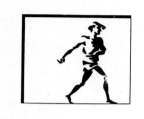

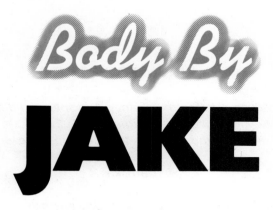

Body By JAKE

by
JAKE STEINFELD

in collaboration with
MELISSA MILLER

Photographs by Nancy Ellison

SIMON AND SCHUSTER
NEW YORK

ACKNOWLEDGEMENTS

The Team: Meliss', "Jefferson", Nancy, and special thanks to my man
"Georgie B."
"The Gang": You know who you are—without you there would be no book
Nike
Caruska
U.C.L.A.
Paul Carafotos—my good buddy and great actor
Thanks to Mary and Ebb for their contribution to Chapter 6

Copyright © 1984 by Body By Jake, Inc.
All rights reserved
including the right of reproduction
in whole or in part in any form
Published by Simon and Schuster
A Division of Simon & Schuster, Inc.
Simon & Schuster Building
Rockefeller Center
1230 Avenue of the Americas
New York, New York, 10020

SIMON AND SCHUSTER and colophon are registered trademarks of Simon & Schuster., Inc.

Designed by — THE TEAM & Robert Walker Advertising

Manufactured in the United States of America
1 2 3 4 5 6 7 8 9 10

Library of Congress Cataloging in Publication Data

Steinfeld, Jake.
Body by Jake.

1. Exercise.   I. Miller, Melissa, 1948-
II. Title.
GV481.S725   1984   613.7'1   84-3909

ISBN 0-671-50321-9

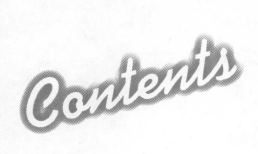

Contents

DEDICATION

My Family
"Grams", Mom and Dad, Andrew, Peter and Nancy

The power of a family is never ending.

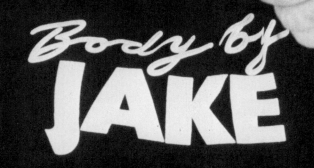

"You don't have to buy a Rolls Royce to own a classy chassis."

Steinfeld '83

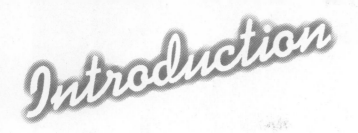

Introduction

Hey! Welcome to Jake's place. Yup, I'm Jake and this is my place or rather my book and these are my exercises and these are my programs and these are my words of advice: if you're going to do something, do it right. And you'll be able to, if you follow my instructions.

These exercises and programs didn't just fall out of the sky and land in this book. I've been an athlete since I was a little kid. (I think I was a little kid for about the first two days after I was born and then I got big….) I changed from team sports to weight training when I was in high school. I couldn't wait for everyone to get it together on the LaCrosse team and with individual exercise I found I only had to answer to me… Jake "The Snake". The more I got into weights the more I got into researching and studying the different ways of working out and finding what works and what doesn't work. I watched people working out at the gym and asked questions. I found out that even though we worked with different weights and with different equipment, we all had something in common: motivation, concentration and the desire to do it right.

I remember, I'd come home from school and go down to the basement to work with my dumbbells. (I learned right away that heavy weights belong in the gym with a spotter watching you.) My Grandma thought I was down in the basement doing my homework. Then my grades came out. My Grandma came down to the basement and told me if I lifted my books as many times as I lifted "those things" I'd be Einstein… oh well.

I didn't end up as Einstein even though I did learn about "mass and velocity". I just thought the only "mass and velocity" I'd ever be interested in would be my own. The idea of being a "personal trainer" never popped up until… (the suspense is killing you?) a friend of mine mentioned that she had a commercial coming up and had to get into better shape pretty fast. I helped her by giving her some basic exercises and running her through them. Even when the commercial had come and gone she kept working out because everyone had started to mention how terrific she looked. The next thing I knew my phone was ringing off the wall with calls from people wanting to get in shape! The first thing I told anyone who called was to go see their doctor first and then call me back. Pretty soon I had clients every day of the week. I loved it. Besides developing my own exercise program I went ahead and adapted it to my different clients. The result is a program that will help you condition your body and lose weight without losing your sense of humor. And, just like I told everybody before you, BEFORE YOU BEGIN ANY KIND OF EXERCISE PROGRAM YOU SHOULD CHECK WITH YOUR DOCTOR AND HAVE HIM DETERMINE WHAT IS BEST FOR YOU!!! Only after this are you ready to start at the beginning of the book. And remember: start ONLY at the beginning!

My form of workout allows you to continually modify your program as you develop strength, stamina, and self-confidence. Whether you're a timid beginner just trying to loosen up, a stressed-out executive releasing tension, a star trying to maintain that "heavenly body" or an advanced weight lifter bench pressing a Plymouth, my program will never take you longer than thirty minutes and has been adapted to fit almost any environment. In other words, this program is for everybody!

So get ready to get down while I take you by the "gluteus maximus" ("tushie") and lead you through my unique exercise book. And just remember, once you start with me, you can never escape. I'm here on every page telling you to "Get lean and mean" "Suck it in" and "No slo' mo"!!!!

Welcome to the team!

Later,

Jake

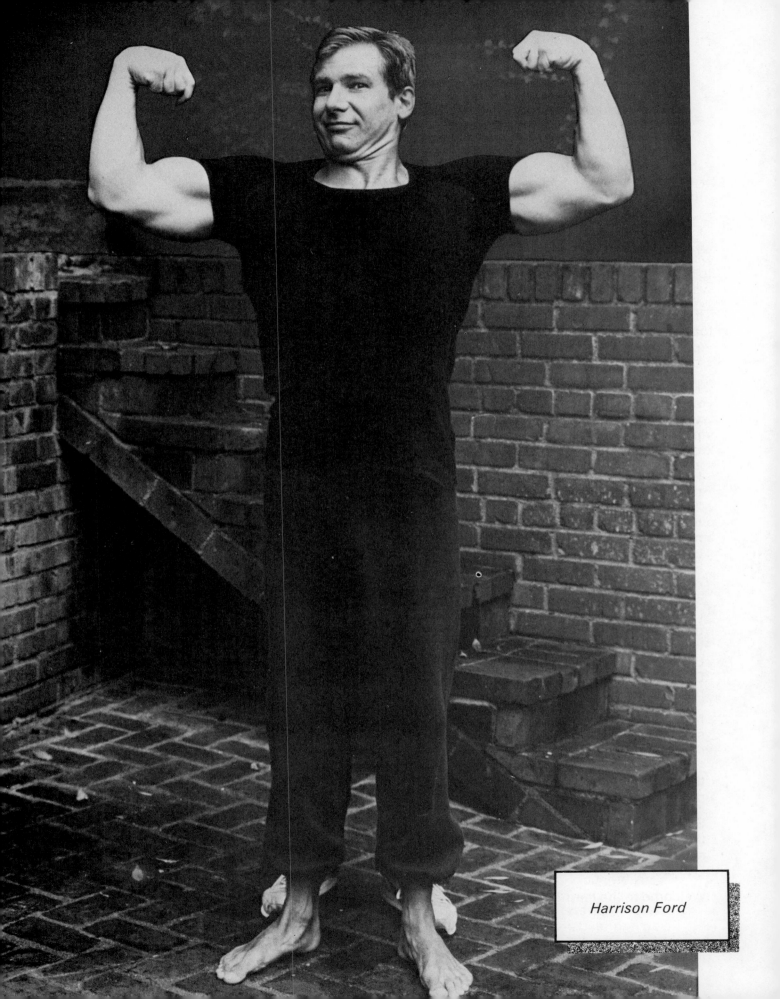

Harrison Ford

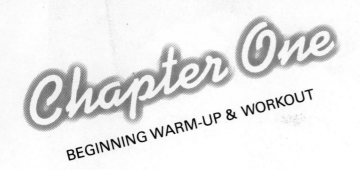

Chapter One

BEGINNING WARM-UP & WORKOUT

Okay all you lemonheads! We gotta get a couple of things straight before we start to train together. Jake "The Snake" here doesn't want you to injure yourself physically or mentally with this workout!

These exercises are designed to improve your general condition by increasing your: muscle tone, strength, endurance, flexibility and heart efficiency. But for any exercises to do this for you, you gotta give yourself a pep talk first. You gotta get yourself really psyched for a truly smokin' workout.

Give yourself a goal!!! You wanna "drop a dime"? Get strong? Maintain what you got? Once you know what your physical goal is, then lock that into your "gray matter". Now your workout will have that motivation to keep it cookin'. BUT, don't set your goals so high that you're defeated before you start. Y'know what I mean? Don't tell yourself, "I'm gonna do 500 'sitters' (sit-ups) by this Friday." It doesn't happen that way, trust me. That's why we're gonna start small.

The workout in this first chapter is the same one I start all my clients with. That's because first we gotta build you some stamina. As you can see, everybody, and I mean EVERYBODY, starts out small. I don't care what exercises you have or haven't done before because I *know* you haven't done these exercises exactly like this. These exercises are listed on the chart and in the explanations in a special order. Keep 'em in just that order!

So, you're gonna start small and you aren't gonna fool around with the order of the exercises. And, one other thing, don't do any big changes in the exercises unless I tell you it's time to or, of course, your doctor tells you. You got two weeks with this first chapter program. And, at the end of these two weeks, if you follow my instructions, you'll feel and see a definite improvement in your physical well-being that'll carry over into your mental well-being. And you also will have become accustomed to the exercises and my own specially developed vocabulary. I mean, if I say "let's go out for some 'lunge'," or "burn it up, and no slo' mo'," "let's cook those 'trimens'," you're not gonna have to stop and look it up! You should also give a look at the body parts chart I've included in this chapter (pp. *12-13*). Not just because it's my body, but because you'll need to know where and what I'm talking about.

This workout will initially take 9 to 12 minutes and, I want you to be totally committed every minute to a full-blown, psyched-out, smokin' workout. Your goal is to do the absolute best you can and keep reaching for that ultimate 30 minute rock 'n rollin' workout doin' the complete number of repetitions in the given amount of time, three times a week!

Are you psyched??? Let's rock 'n roll. Here's what you need:
>   sneakers
>   sweat suit (and I want you to SWEAT!)
>   towel
>   broomstick
>   one clock with a second hand so you can time the exercises the first couple of
>   workouts and get the feel of working at top speed.

First, be an egghead and learn the body parts and the vocabulary.

Anatomy By Jake

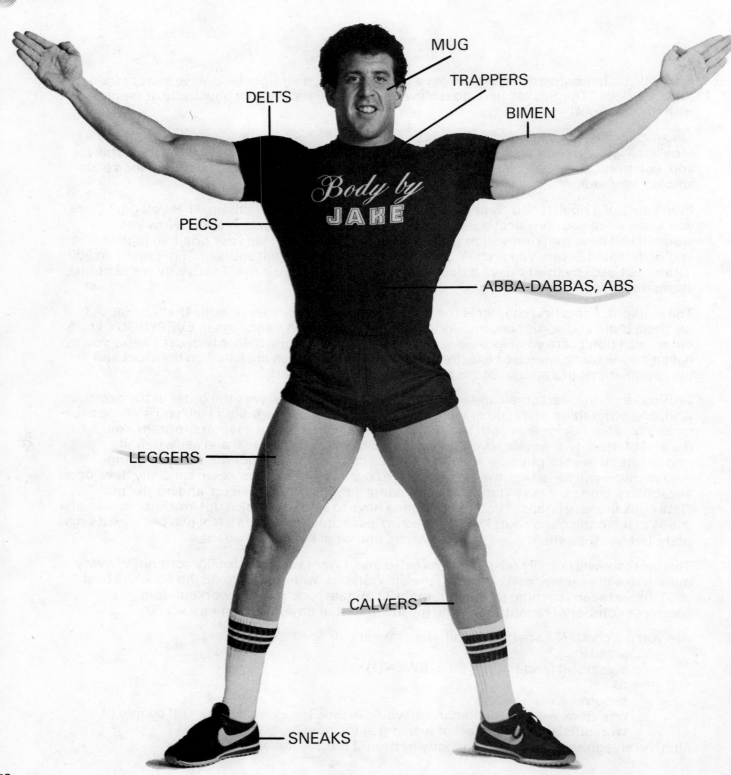

MUG

TRAPPERS

DELTS

BIMEN

Body by JAKE

PECS

ABBA-DABBAS, ABS

LEGGERS

CALVERS

SNEAKS

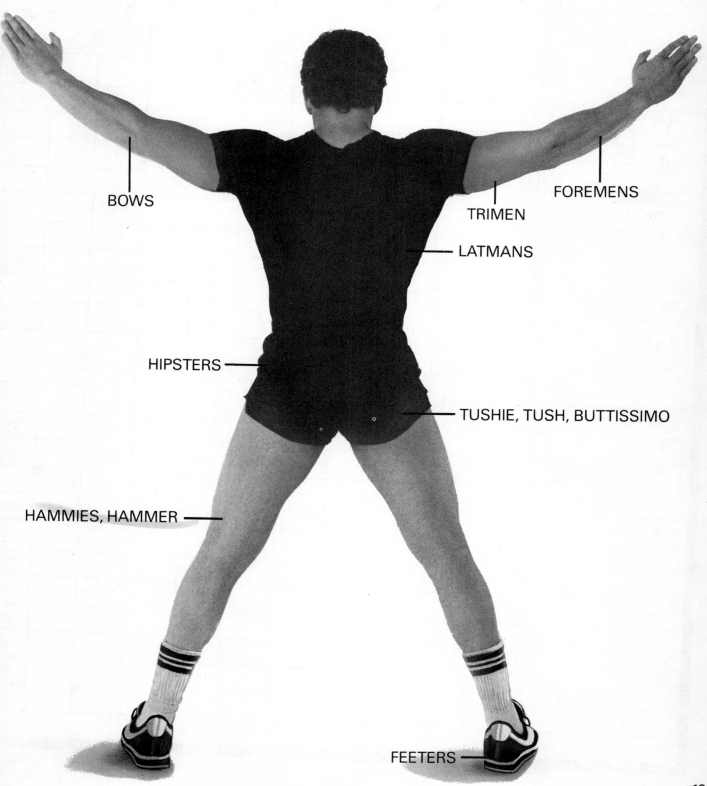

BOWS

FOREMENS

TRIMEN

LATMANS

HIPSTERS

TUSHIE, TUSH, BUTTISSIMO

HAMMIES, HAMMER

FEETERS

13

BEGINNING WARM-UP & WORKOUT

- READ EACH EXERCISE CAREFULLY! TRY SLOWLY! PUSH YOURSELF GENTLY!
- REPS ARE *SUGGESTED* NUMBERS
- 1 WORKOUT AT EACH LEVEL IF POSSIBLE
- THIS PROGRAM IS 3 WORKOUTS A WEEK FOR 2 WEEKS

CHAPTER ONE

EXERCISES	Workout 1 REPS	U DID	Workout 2 REPS	U DID	Workout 3 REPS	U DID	Workout 4 REPS	U DID	Workout 5 REPS	U DID	GOAL
BIG STRETCH	5		3		3		4		4		5
HEAD ROLLS (each direction)	5		5		5		5		5		5
ARM CIRCLES (each direction)	30		32		32		34		34		35
TWISTERS (full twist one count)	30		32		32		34		34		35
BROOMSTICK: TWISTERS	30				17		18		19		20
SIDE STRETCHES	15		16		17		18		19		20
SINGLE SIDE STRETCHES	15		16		17		18		19		35
BENT OVER TWISTERS	30		31		32		33		34		10
SIDE: STRETCHES	10		10		10		10		10		10
SINGLES	10		10		10		10		10		10
OVERHEAD	10		10		10		10		10		5
SINGLE OVERHEAD	1		(HOLD FOR 15 COUNTS—EACH SIDE)								20
TOE TOUCHES	15		16		17		18		19		20
RUN #1	15		16		17		18		19		20
BUTT BURNERS #1 (Women) (each side)	15		16		17		18		19		10
PUSH-UPS #1 (Men)	5		6		7		8		9		20
RUNS #2	15		16		17		18		19		20
BUTT BURNERS #2 (each side)	15		16		17		18		19		10
PUSH-UPS #2	5		6		7		8		9		20
SIT-UPS	15		16		17		18		19		20
LEG RAISES— IN/OUTS	15		16		17		18		19		20
SCISSORS	15		16		17		18		19		20
BABY RUNS	15		16		17		18		19		20
RUNS #3	15		16		17		18		19		20

EXERCISES	Workout 1 REPS	U DID	Workout 2 REPS	DID	Workout 3 REPS	DID	Workout 4 REPS	DID	Workout 5 REPS	DID	GOAL
BUTT BURNERS #3 (each side)	15		16		17		18		19		20
PUSH-UPS #3	5		6		7		8		9		10
PUSH-UPS (all)	5		6/10		7/10		8/15		9/15		10/20
OVER HEAD STRETCH	1		(HOLD FOR 15 COUNTS—EACH SIDE)								2
DOOR KNOB CURLS	10		11		12		13		14		15
TRICEP PUSH-UP	5		6		7		8		9		15
RUNS #4	15		16		17		18		19		20
BUTT BURNERS #4 (Women) each side	15		16		17		18		19		20
PUSH-UPS #4 (Men)	5		6		7		8		9		10
LUNGES (each side)	10		11		12		13		14		15
WISHBONE STRETCH	1		(HOLD FOR 15 COUNTS—EACH SIDE)								1
HURDLES	1		(HOLD FOR 15 COUNTS—EACH SIDE)								1
EGG ROLLS	1		(HOLD FOR 15 COUNTS)								1

Jake Jargon

abs, abba-dabbas—abdomen
baby sitters—sit-ups
bimen—bicep
bonus—extra good
get psyched—to get in the right frame of mind
gettin' hot—to begin to catch on
hammies—hamstrings
hurts—hurdle stretch
hustle—to move fast and not stop
light 'em up—to use enough energy to promote spontaneous combustion
lungeroos, lungarrows—lunges
max—maximum
pecs—pectoral—chest muscles located between collarbone and breastbone
rep—one complete movement of exercises is called a repetition
rock 'em—same as "hustle"
sets—number of reps done consecutively from start to finish
sitters—sit-ups
slo' mo'—slow motion
smokin'—immediately following "gettin' hot"
sneaks—sneakers, gym shoes
streamlined—keeping back flat, tushie down and legs stretched out for runs
sweats—sweat suit
trimen—tricep
tush,tushie—buttocks, fanny, bottom
twisteroos—exercise know as Twisters
x's—times

Now that we speak the same language, go through all the exercises carefully and read every instruction and look at every picture and be sure you have the right form. The number of reps is your starting number. Look at the exercise chart *before* you continue working out to see how many to add and when so you'll know your goal.

Are you psyched? Well, let's hustle then. Maybe we can even light 'em up by the end of this chapter.

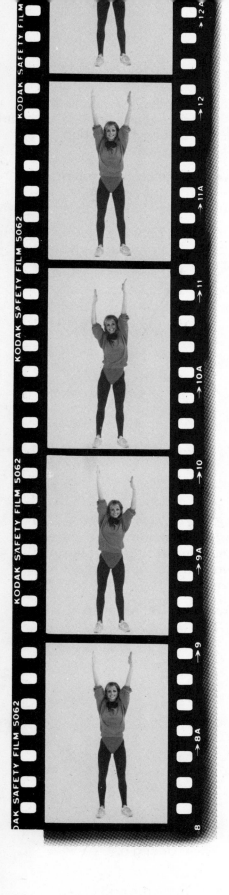

Big Stretch

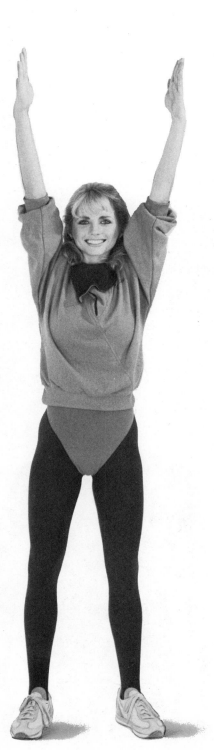

FOR: Loosening up arms, middle back and waist
REPS: 5x's each side, alternating sides
TIME: 10 seconds altogether

Take this real slow and feel your body start to loosen. Then feel it get warm and then get ready to get truly HOT!

1. Stand straight, shoulders back, feet shoulder width apart and your arms raised straight up above your head with your palms facing each other.

2. Alternately reach each arm in the air as far as it will go, keeping your elbows by your ears, five times for each arm.

Reach for it, "partner"! And, get ready to move a little faster real soon ... like as soon as you turn the page!

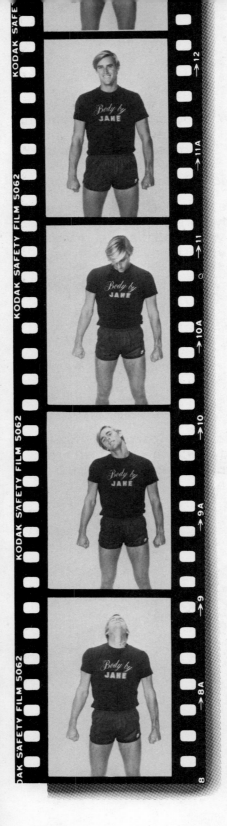

Head Rolls

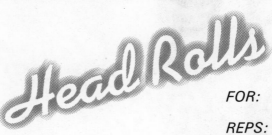

FOR: Loosening up and getting ready for a smokin' workout
REPS: 5x's each direction
TIME: 15 seconds

We're gonna rock 'n roll right after this but, right now, we're just gonna roll.

This is the only exercise we're ever gonna do slow! Take advantage of it!

1. *Stand straight, shoulders back, feet shoulder width apart, arms straight down at your sides, fists clenched and EVERYTHING HELD FLEXED AND TIGHT!!!*

2. *Squeeze your "tushie" together as tight as you can while holding your stomach in and slowly drop your chin on your chest.*

3. *Slowly roll your head around in a complete circle five times <u>in one direction</u> and then five times in the <u>opposite direction</u>.*

KEEP YOUR BODY NICE AND TIGHT! Remember to always keep everything tight during the workout no matter what level you are.

Aw right! Get ready to hustle!

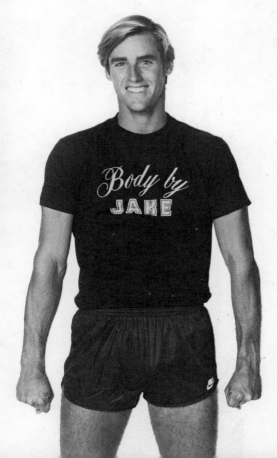

Arm Circles

FOR: Warming up the upper body, strengthening upper back and chest, gettin' your heart pumpin'!!

REPS: 30x's each direction

TIME: 10 seconds in each direction

Okay, let's get rockin'! It's time to pick up speed and never, ever quit! You gotta get psyched! Let's light em' up! Concentrate on keepin' everything real tight!

1. *Stand with feet shoulder width apart, knees slightly bent, and extend your arms straight out from your shoulders with fists clenched. Squeeze your "tushie" real tight, flex the stomach real tight.*

2. *Rotate your arms in small circles from the shoulders keeping everything nice and TIGHT!*

Keep 'em rollin'! You got 10 seconds to do 30 in one direction and 10 seconds to do 30 in the opposite direction.

So gimme 30 in each direction.

FEEL IT BURN UP IN YOUR SHOULDERS! DON''T SLOW DOWN!!!

Gettin' warm? Great!

Let's get to Twisters!

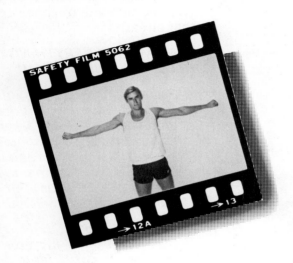

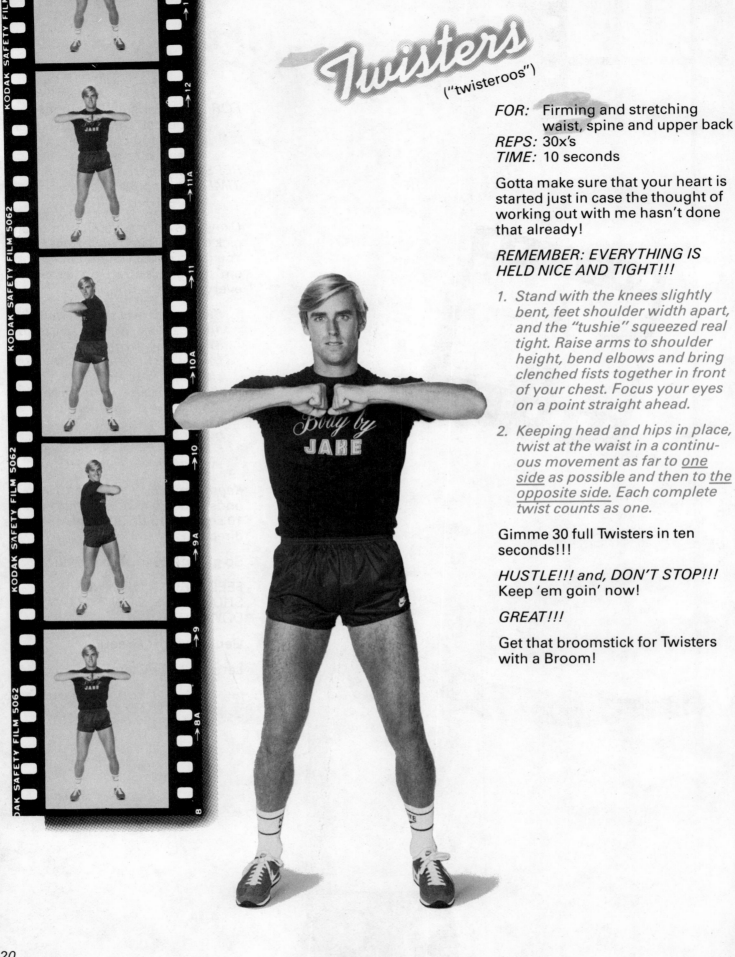

Twisters

("twisteroos")

FOR: Firming and stretching
waist, spine and upper back

REPS: 30x's

TIME: 10 seconds

Gotta make sure that your heart is started just in case the thought of working out with me hasn't done that already!

REMEMBER: EVERYTHING IS HELD NICE AND TIGHT!!!

1. *Stand with the knees slightly bent, feet shoulder width apart, and the "tushie" squeezed real tight. Raise arms to shoulder height, bend elbows and bring clenched fists together in front of your chest. Focus your eyes on a point straight ahead.*

2. *Keeping head and hips in place, twist at the waist in a continuous movement as far to one side as possible and then to the opposite side. Each complete twist counts as one.*

Gimme 30 full Twisters in ten seconds!!!

HUSTLE!!! and, DON'T STOP!!! Keep 'em goin' now!

GREAT!!!

Get that broomstick for Twisters with a Broom!

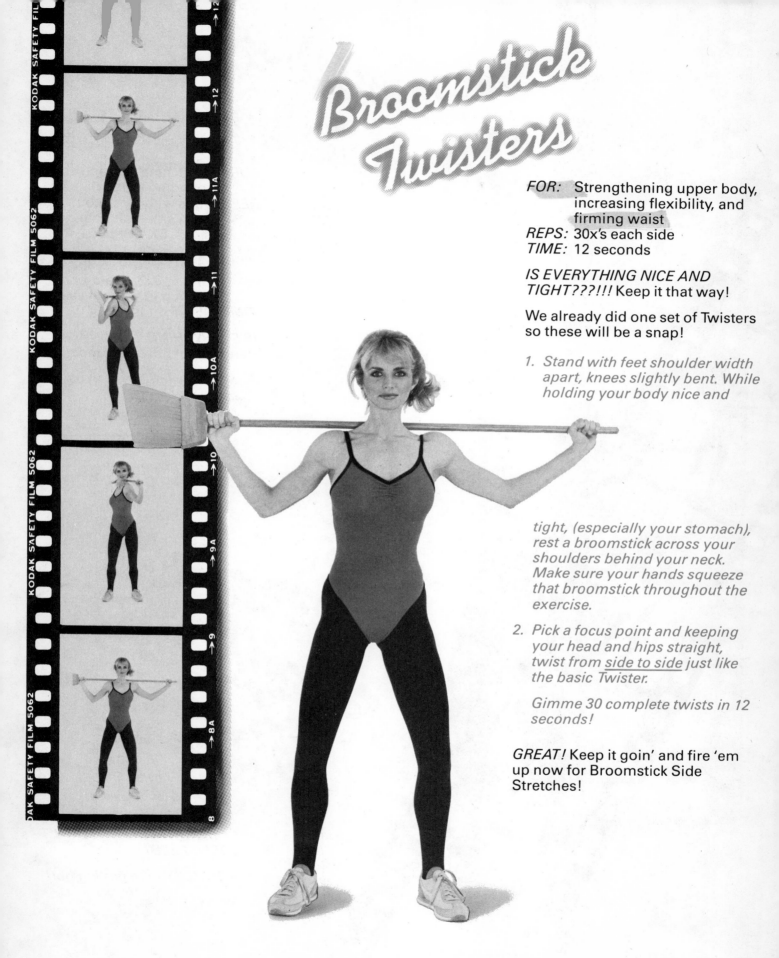

Broomstick Twisters

FOR: Strengthening upper body, increasing flexibility, and firming waist

REPS: 30x's each side

TIME: 12 seconds

IS EVERYTHING NICE AND TIGHT???!!! Keep it that way!

We already did one set of Twisters so these will be a snap!

1. *Stand with feet shoulder width apart, knees slightly bent. While holding your body nice and tight, (especially your stomach), rest a broomstick across your shoulders behind your neck. Make sure your hands squeeze that broomstick throughout the exercise.*

2. *Pick a focus point and keeping your head and hips straight, twist from <u>side to side</u> just like the basic Twister.*

   Gimme 30 complete twists in 12 seconds!

GREAT! Keep it goin' and fire 'em up now for Broomstick Side Stretches!

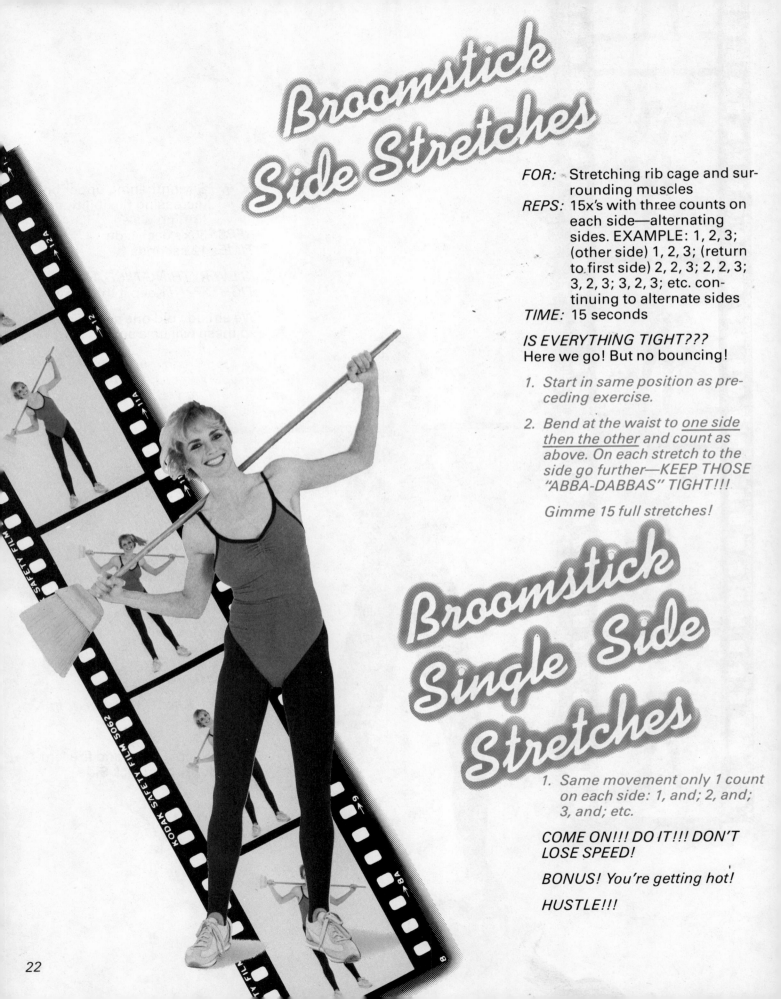

Broomstick Side Stretches

FOR: Stretching rib cage and surrounding muscles

REPS: 15x's with three counts on each side—alternating sides. EXAMPLE: 1, 2, 3; (other side) 1, 2, 3; (return to first side) 2, 2, 3; 2, 2, 3; 3, 2, 3; 3, 2, 3; etc. continuing to alternate sides

TIME: 15 seconds

IS EVERYTHING TIGHT???
Here we go! But no bouncing!

1. Start in same position as preceding exercise.

2. Bend at the waist to <u>one side then the other</u> and count as above. On each stretch to the side go further—KEEP THOSE "ABBA-DABBAS" TIGHT!!!

Gimme 15 full stretches!

Broomstick Single Side Stretches

1. Same movement only 1 count on each side: 1, and; 2, and; 3, and; etc.

COME ON!!! DO IT!!! DON'T LOSE SPEED!

BONUS! You're getting hot!

HUSTLE!!!

Bent Over Broomstick Twisters

FOR: Stretching waist, spine, chest, shoulders, upper back, hamstrings
REPS: 30x's each side
TIME: 15 seconds

Okay, this is it for the broomstick stuff so LIGHT 'EM UP!

Is EVERYTHING tight???

These are just like the Broomstick Twisters only you're bent over from the waist with a flat back.

1. *Keeping the broomstick where it is, bend over from the waist with the knees slightly bent and your back flat.*

2. *Twist from <u>side to side</u> as far as you can trying to bring the end of the broom as close to leg as possible.*

   Gimme 30 full Twisters in 15 seconds.

ROCK 'EM AND GO! GO! GO!

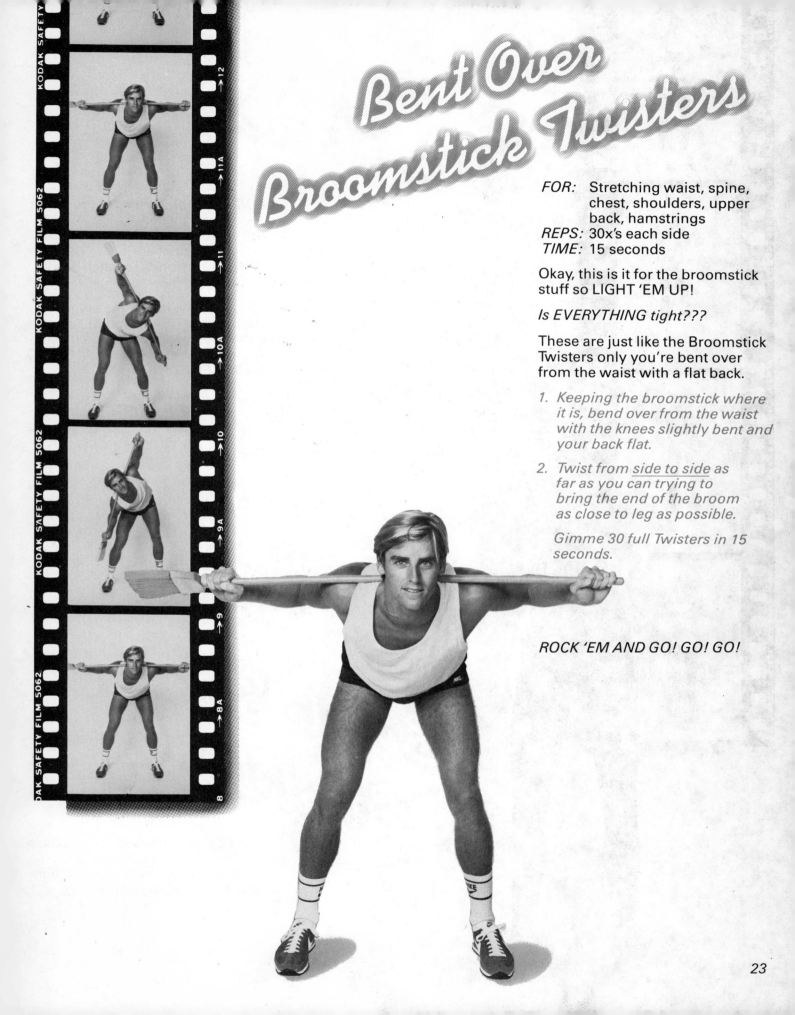

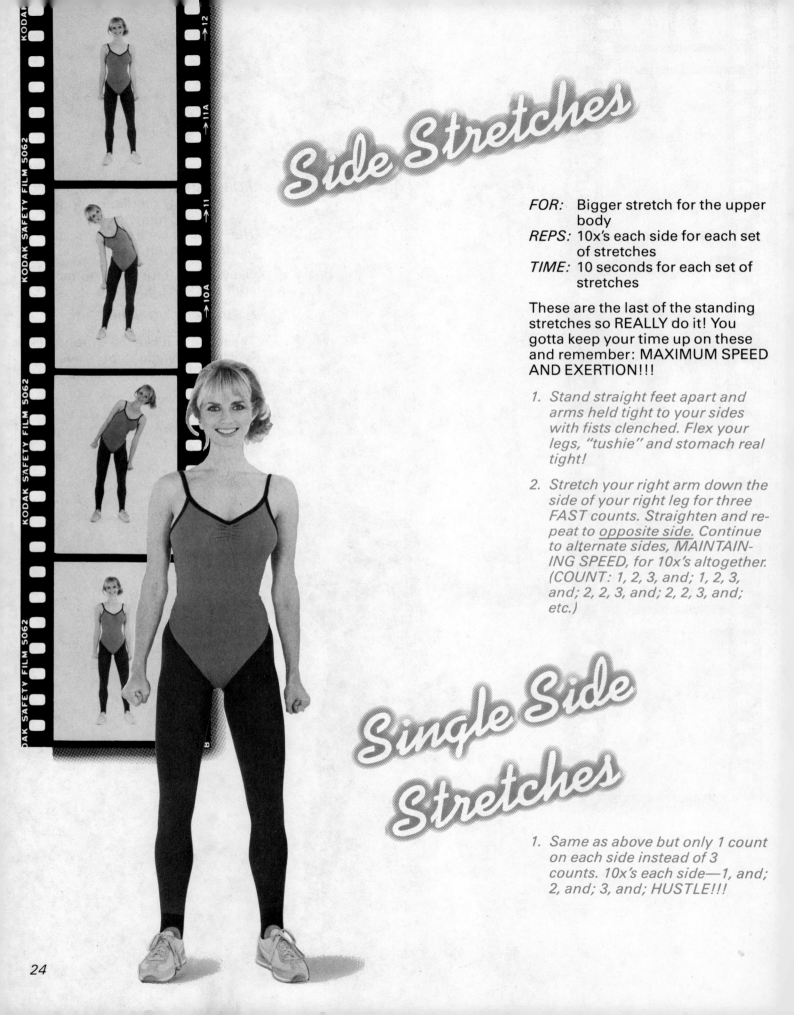

Side Stretches

FOR: Bigger stretch for the upper body
REPS: 10x's each side for each set of stretches
TIME: 10 seconds for each set of stretches

These are the last of the standing stretches so REALLY do it! You gotta keep your time up on these and remember: MAXIMUM SPEED AND EXERTION!!!

1. Stand straight feet apart and arms held tight to your sides with fists clenched. Flex your legs, "tushie" and stomach real tight!

2. Stretch your right arm down the side of your right leg for three FAST counts. Straighten and repeat to opposite side. Continue to alternate sides, MAINTAINING SPEED, for 10x's altogether. (COUNT: 1, 2, 3, and; 1, 2, 3, and; 2, 2, 3, and; 2, 2, 3, and; etc.)

Single Side Stretches

1. Same as above but only 1 count on each side instead of 3 counts. 10x's each side—1, and; 2, and; 3, and; HUSTLE!!!

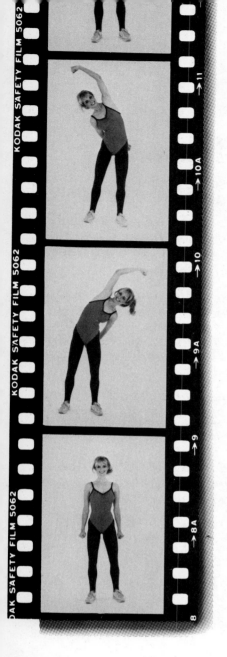

Over Head Side Stretches

1. Stand with feet apart, arms at sides with fists clenched. Raise right arm over your head with elbow slightly bent and bend your left arm behind your waist with fist clenched.

2. Stretch to your left side for 3 fast counts alternating sides as before: (1, 2, 3; 1, 2, 3; 2, 2, 3; 2, 2, 3; etc.). Both sides together are one count.

3. Alternating sides, gimme 10 full OVER HEAD SIDE STRETCHES!

Single Over Head Side Stretches

1. Same starting position as above.

2. Lean to one side holding stretch for 15 counts, and then to opposite side. DON'T BOUNCE!

1x on each side.

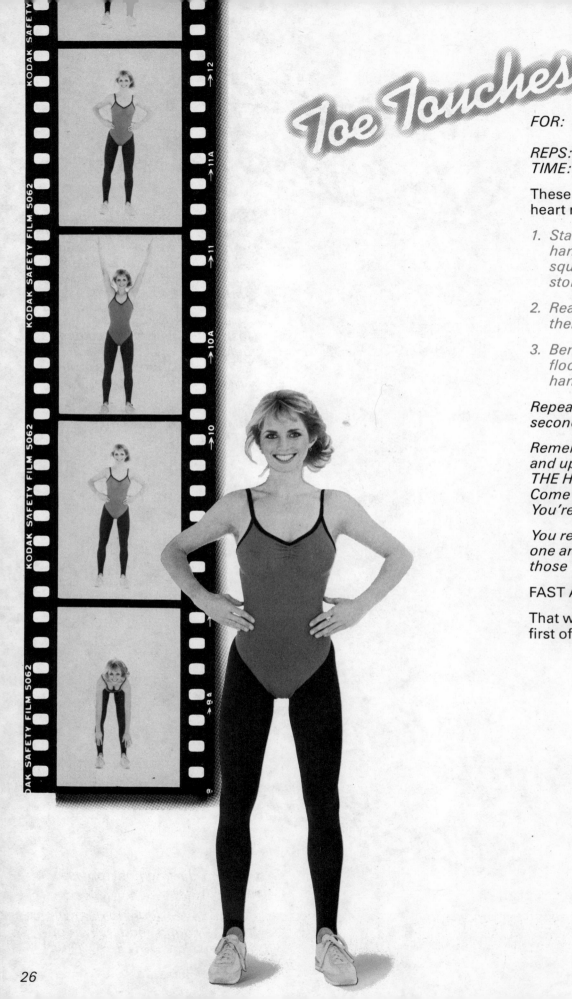

Toe Touches

FOR: Stretching hamstrings and arms
REPS: 15x's
TIME: 20 seconds

These are guaranteed to get your heart rate up to the MAX!!!

1. *Stand with feet apart and with hands on hips. Flex the legs, squeeze the butt, flex the stomach real tight!*

2. *Reach both arms straight up then return hands to hips.*

3. *Bend at waist and reach for the floor. Straighten and return hands to hips.*

Repeat steps 2 and 3 15x's in 30 seconds!!!

Remember the form: touch hips and up, touch hips and down. THE HIPS ARE HOME BASE! Come on, let's keep it smokin'! You're halfway there!!!

You really gotta hustle on this one and feel that stretch in those "hammies."

FAST AS YOU CAN!!!

That was BONUS!!! Let's go for the first of the "Steinfeld Sprints"!

Runs #1

FOR: Maintaining cardio-vascular level while working arms, back, stomach, legs, calves and feet

REPS: 15x's (There are 4 sets of these spaced throughout the workout)

TIME: 7 seconds

These are the famous "Steinfeld Sprints" that my clients love so much. You gotta get your form right from the very beginning. Follow the instructions very carefully and NO JOGGING!!! You gotta sprint!

DOWN ON THE FLOOR! (at last)

1. *Support yourself on your hands and toes as though you were doing Push-ups—but with one leg extended straight out and the other flexed toward your chest. Keeping your "tushie" down, try to be STREAMLINED!*

2. *Alternate legs as if running in place, bring one knee all the way up to your chest with the other leg extended and then alternate legs and continue running while supporting yourself on your hands.*

3. *Each right and left together is 1 count. So, count 1, and; 2, and; up to 15 and gimme 15 in 7 seconds!*

GO! GO! GO! GO! GO! GO! GO! GO! GO! GO! GO! GO! GO! GO! GO! GO! SPRINT! SPRINT! SPRINT! SPRINT! SPRINT! SPRINT! SPRINT! SPRINT!

That's it! You got it! Keep it smokin'!

Stay down there for Butt Burners! Ladies Only!

Gentlemen! You're always gonna do Push-ups when the ladies do Butt Burners!

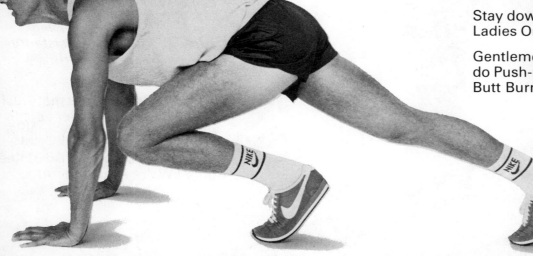

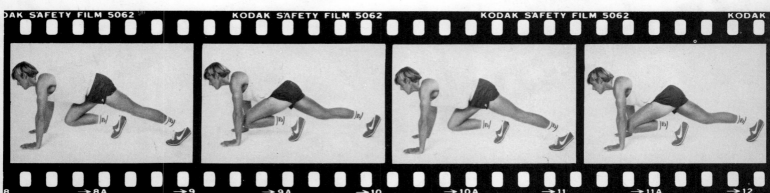

Butt Burners #1

FOR: GUESS!
REPS: 15x's each leg. (There are 4 sets of these spaced throughout the workout)
TIME: 15 seconds each leg

Don't think you get to rest! Read this fast and get ready for Butt Burners!

You have to use yourself as resistance in raising and lowering your leg. Just pretend I'm there exerting pressure on that leg as you try to raise it.

So let's do Butt Burners and remember to "resist yourself"... I know it's hard.

1. *On hands and knees, extend the right leg directly out behind you with toes pointing down.*

2. *Keeping your back flat, raise your extended leg and then lower it to the starting position, trying to get it higher each time you raise it.*

KEEP EVERYTHING TIGHT IN CASE YOU'VE FORGOTTEN!!!

Gimme 15 reps on each leg adding a little more resistance with each rep. FEEL THE PRESSURE.

Work that leg and feel that "tushie" get smaller and smaller as it BURNS!

Get 'em up! Come on! Do it! Keep it goin'! We're almost there!

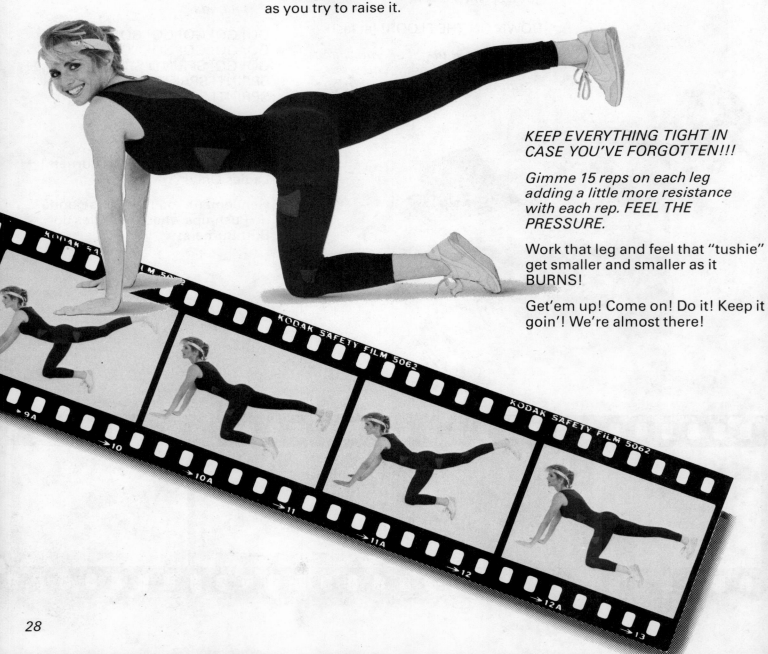

28

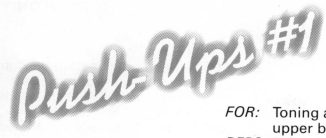

Push-Ups #1

FOR: Toning and strengthening upper body
REPS: 5x's
TIME: 5 seconds

Maybe you've never done this kind before but don't think just because you bend your knees and don't touch your chin to the floor that they're easy.

1. *Get down on your hands and knees.*

2. *Bend your elbows and roll forward on your knees, lowering your chest towards the floor and then push yourself back to starting position.*

Do these very rapidly and keep that fanny and stomach TIGHT!

Gimme 5! And I don't mean a handshake!

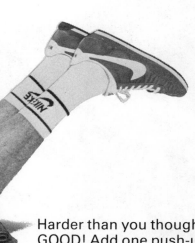

Harder than you thought???
GOOD! Add one push-up at your next workout!

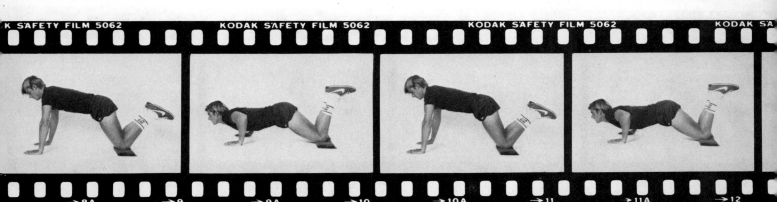

Runs #2

FOR: Maintaining cardio-vascular level while working arms, back, stomach, legs, calves, feet

REPS: 15x's (Both legs together is one count)

TIME: 7 seconds

Okay lemonheads! Watch your form! Don't jog! No slo' mo'!

1. *Support yourself on your hands and toes as though you were doing Push-ups—but with one leg extended straight out and the other flexed toward your chest. Keeping your "tushie" down, try to be STREAMLINED!*

2. *Alternate legs as if running in place, bring one knee all the way up to your chest with the other leg extended and then alternate legs and continue running while supporting yourself on your hands.*

3. *Each right and left together is 1 count. So count 1, and; 2, and; up to 15 and gimme 15 in 7 seconds!*

   You gotta maintain your speed in order to build stamina!!!

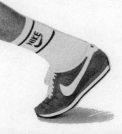

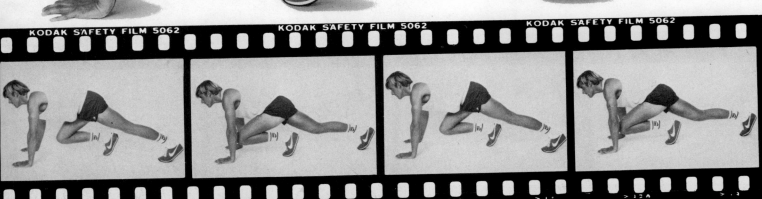

Butt Burners #2

FOR: You know!
REPS: 15x's each leg. This is the second set of 4
TIME: 15 seconds each leg

You gotta gimme enough resistance on this one so that you feel it burn!

1. On hands and knees as shown, extend right leg directly out behind you with foot pointed down.

   KEEP EVERYTHING TIGHT IN CASE YOU'VE FORGOTTEN!

2. Raise and lower your leg trying to get it higher each time. Feel the pressure and gimme 15 <u>on each leg</u>. NO RESTING!!!

Did you burn it out! BONUS!!! Let's do some "sitters"!

By the way, you're doing great if you've even gotten this far on your first day!

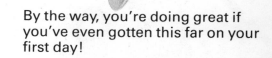

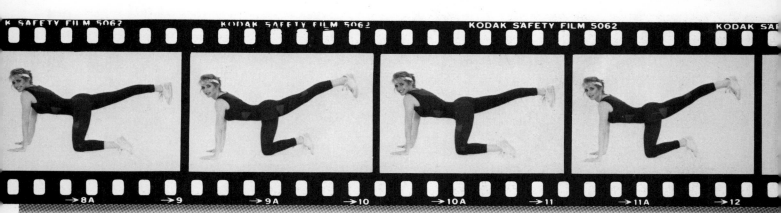

Push-Ups #2

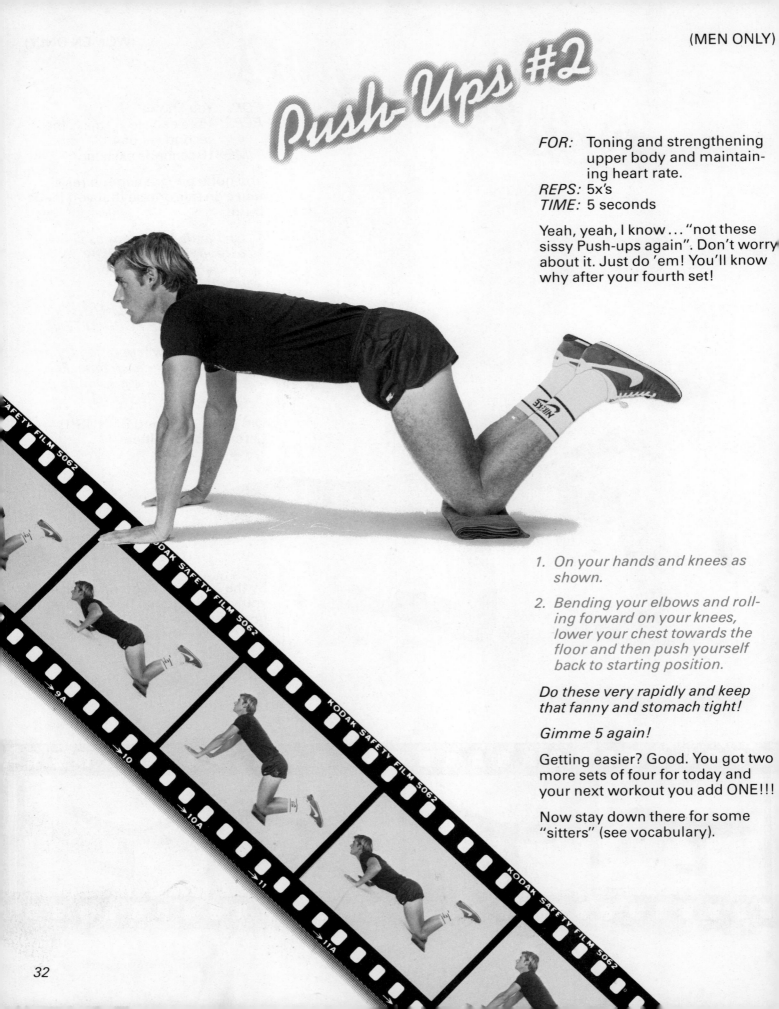

FOR: Toning and strengthening upper body and maintaining heart rate.
REPS: 5x's
TIME: 5 seconds

Yeah, yeah, I know... "not these sissy Push-ups again". Don't worry about it. Just do 'em! You'll know why after your fourth set!

1. On your hands and knees as shown.

2. Bending your elbows and rolling forward on your knees, lower your chest towards the floor and then push yourself back to starting position.

Do these very rapidly and keep that fanny and stomach tight!

Gimme 5 again!

Getting easier? Good. You got two more sets of four for today and your next workout you add ONE!!!

Now stay down there for some "sitters" (see vocabulary).

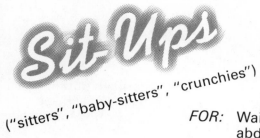

Sit-Ups

("sitters", "baby-sitters", "crunchies")

FOR: Waist, upper and lower abdomen ("abs", "abba-dabbas", etc.)
REPS: 15 x's
TIME: 15 seconds

These are not, I repeat, are not the Sit-ups like you did in junior high school. These are done with your legs bent and will make you scream out for mercy the first couple of workouts. BUT they will become easier real fast!

Your goal is 15 reps. If you can't do 15...do as many as you can. When you think you can't even do one more... GIMME ONE MORE! One last thing pea-brains: FAT DEPOSITS AROUND YOUR "ABBA-DABBAS" ARE WHAT MAKE THIS EXERCISE SO HARD!!! Think about it.

1. *Lie on the floor with your knees bent and feet flat on the floor, arms stretched out in front with palms facing each other.*

2. *Lift your head high enough to bring shoulder blades off the floor, and reach your hands between your knees. Relax to starting position. Gimme as many of these as you can towards 15.*

Stay down on the floor for more stomach work.

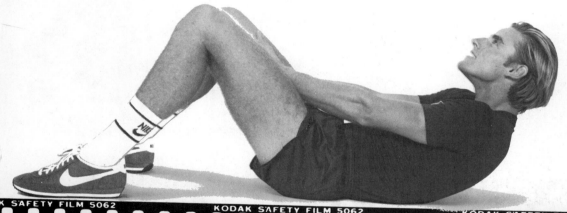

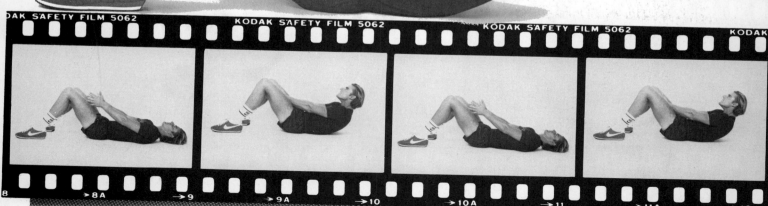

Leg Raises

FOR: Stomach and thighs
REPS: 15x's for each set
TIME: 15 seconds for each set

These three exercises must be done together! And, you'd better not stop in between! Got me? We're gonna do In/Outs, Scissors, and Baby Runs; all on your back in the same position.

In/Outs

1. Lie flat on your back with your hands under your "tushie" and your head raised.

2. Bring your knees in to your chest and push them straight out again, keeping your feet a few inches off the floor.

3. Repeat by pulling knees up to chest again and pushing out.

   Gimme a smokin' 15 and go on to Scissors as shown. Remember—don't let your feet touch the floor during or between the exercises!

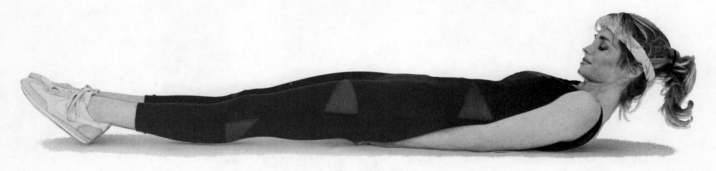

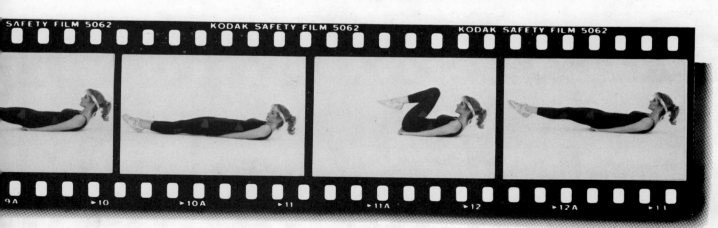

34

Scissors

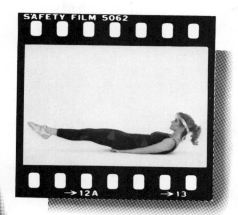

1. Next 15: legs extended straight out parallel to the floor and held tight.

2. Cross legs back and forth, left over right and right over left, as shown for 15 and, GET TOUGH!

Baby Runs

1. Last 15: holding legs straight and TIGHT, flutter stiff legs in tiny runs for 15 counts.

DON'T EVER LET ME CATCH YOU WITH YOUR FEET NEAR THE FLOOR DURING THIS EXERCISE!!!!

Aw right! It's time to get lean and mean for another 15 runs!

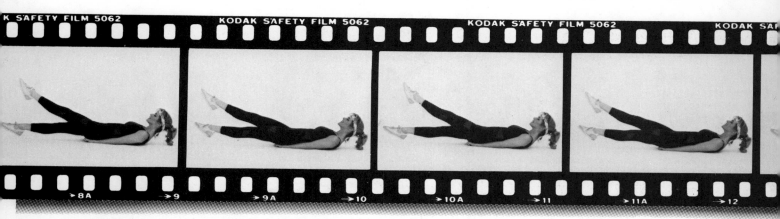

Runs #3

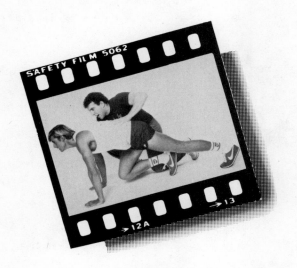

FOR: Maintaining cardio-vascular level while working arms, back, stomach, legs, calves and feet

REPS: 15x's (This is the third set of 4)

TIME: 7 seconds

Do you know what to do??? You gotta GET DOWN!

1. *Support yourself on your hands and toes as though you were doing Push-ups—but with one leg extended straight out and the other flexed toward your chest. Keeping your "tushie" down, try to be STREAMLINED!*

2. *Alternate legs as if running in place, bring opposite knee all the way up to your chest as you extend the other leg and continue running while supporting yourself on your hands.*

Legs together, 1 count!
GO FOR IT!!!

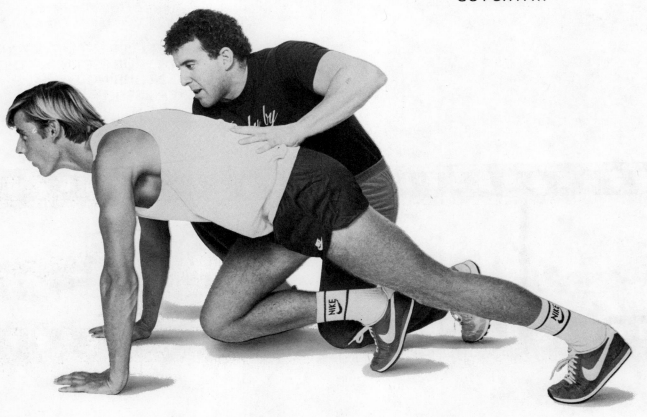

Butt Burners #3

FOR: "Tushies" around the world
REPS: 15x's each leg. This is the third set of 4.
TIME: 15 seconds each leg.

This is your next to the last time to try and work your butt off! Literally . . .

1. On hands and knees as shown with right leg extended directly out behind you, foot pointed down.

2. Keep everything held TIGHT, and raise and lower your leg trying to get it higher each time.

3. Resisting yourself, gimme 15 on each leg and SMOKE IT!!!

Let's do some work on that upper body.

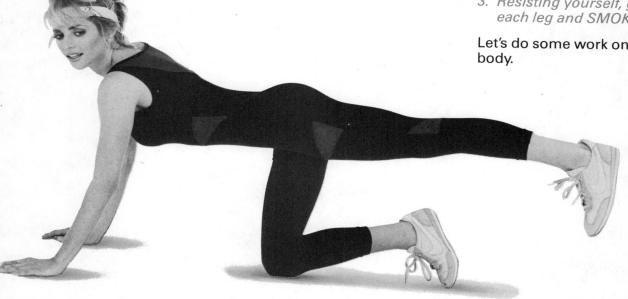

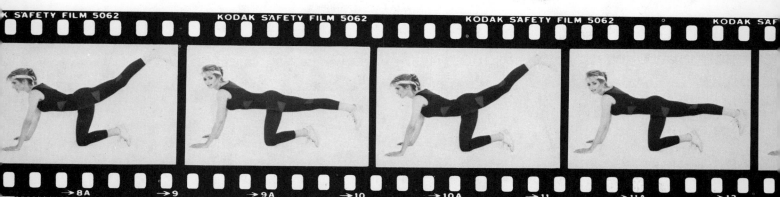

Push-Ups #3

FOR: Toning and strengthening upper body and maintaining heart rate
REPS: 5x's
TIME: 15 seconds

Gettin' a little winded? Good! Then you're smokin.' So, keep your time up and keep hustling!

1. On your hands and knees as before.

2. Bending your elbows and rolling forward on your knees, lower your chest towards the floor and then push yourself back to starting position.

Do these fast, fast, fast and hold that stomach and fanny tight, tight, tight.

Gimme a smokin' 5!

Don't quit! Keep goin'. I gotta surprise for you on the next page.

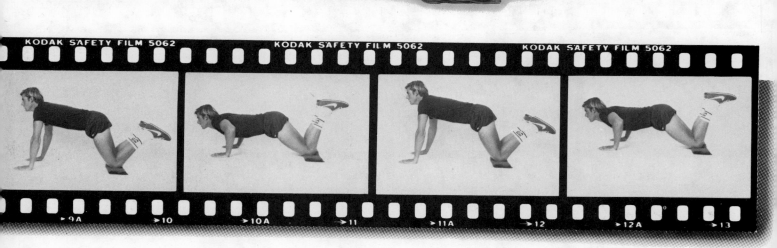

Push-Ups

FOR: Toning and strengthening upper body and maintaining heart rate
REPS: 5x's
TIME: 15 seconds

Okay fellas, these should be a snap for you! Ladies, read these instructions carefully since you've never done these before.

1. *On your hands and knees.*

2. *Bending your elbows and rolling forward on your knees, lower your chest towards the floor and then push yourself back to starting position.*

Do these very rapidly and keep that fanny and stomach tight!!!

Gimme 5!

Go for it!!!

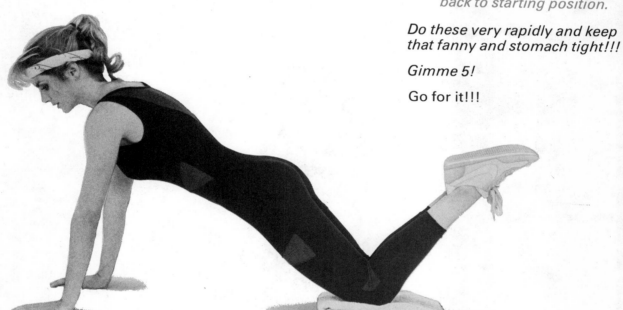

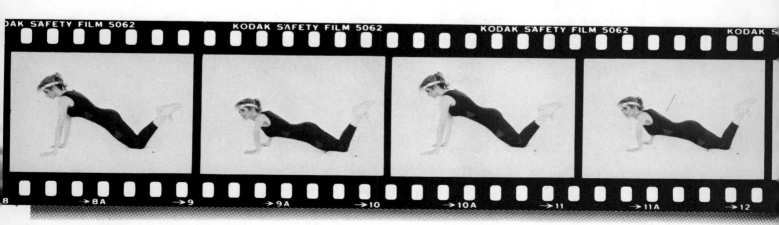

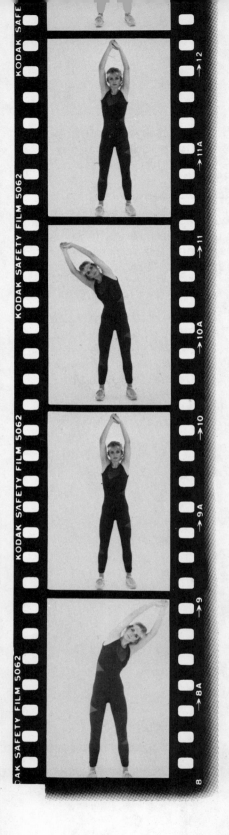

Over Head Stretch

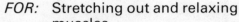

FOR: Stretching out and relaxing muscles

REPS: Hold for 15 counts—ONCE in each position

TIME: 30 seconds

1. *Stand straight feet apart with everything held tight and hands clasped straight above head.*

2. *Bend to one side feeling the stretch along your rib cage. Straighten up and bend to opposite side. HOLD FOR 15 SECONDS <u>on each side.</u>*

That's it! Feel good? It should. Now don't try and escape out that door—we got a little more work, sport!

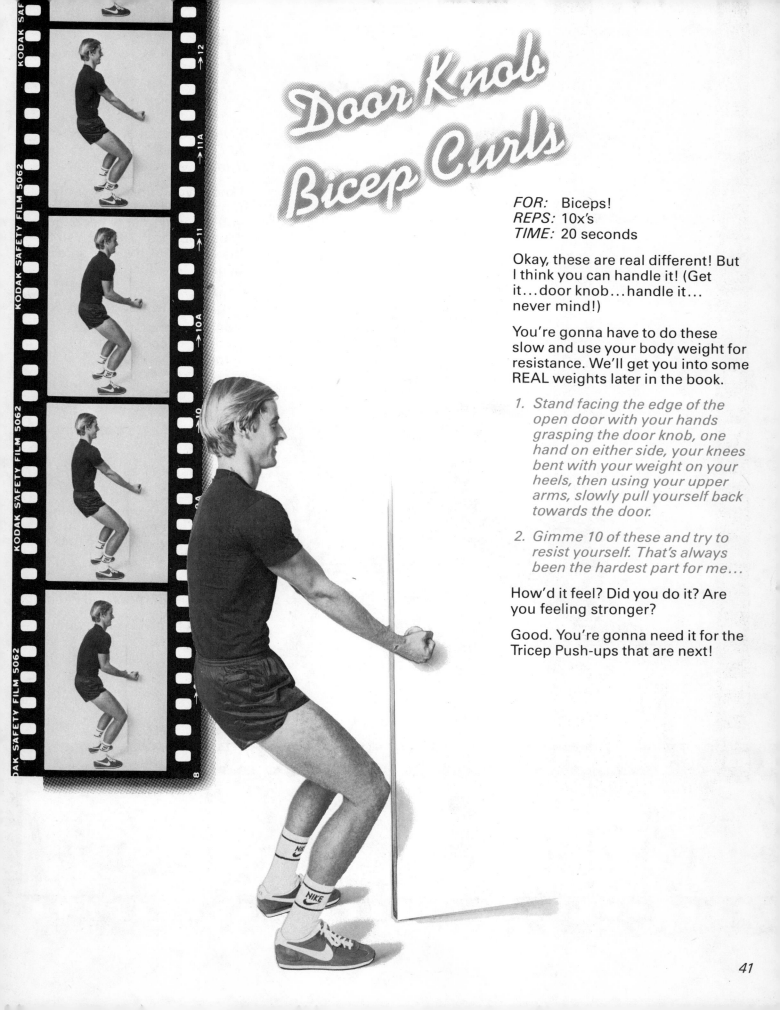

Door Knob Bicep Curls

FOR: Biceps!
REPS: 10x's
TIME: 20 seconds

Okay, these are real different! But I think you can handle it! (Get it…door knob…handle it… never mind!)

You're gonna have to do these slow and use your body weight for resistance. We'll get you into some REAL weights later in the book.

1. *Stand facing the edge of the open door with your hands grasping the door knob, one hand on either side, your knees bent with your weight on your heels, then using your upper arms, slowly pull yourself back towards the door.*

2. *Gimme 10 of these and try to resist yourself. That's always been the hardest part for me…*

How'd it feel? Did you do it? Are you feeling stronger?

Good. You're gonna need it for the Tricep Push-ups that are next!

41

Tricep Push-Up

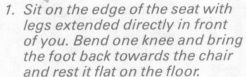

("trimens")

FOR: Backs of upper arms
REPS: 5x's
TIME: 10 seconds

I know, you think, "gee, only 5 reps"! You'll see why! And I want you to remember to keep those "abba-dabbas" TIGHT! You'll need the edge of a chair, the sofa or a bench.

1. Sit on the edge of the seat with legs extended directly in front of you. Bend one knee and bring the foot back towards the chair and rest it flat on the floor.

2. Grip the edge of the chair and raise your buttocks off the seat and slowly lower yourself towards the floor and then return to starting position.

3. Gimme 5 big ones up and down. And keep it smooth!

After that I bet you're looking forward to some Runs! You never thought you'd ever see that day, did you?

Aw right! Let's do one last set of Runs, Butt Burners and Push-ups.

One last thing…you're doin' GREAT!!!

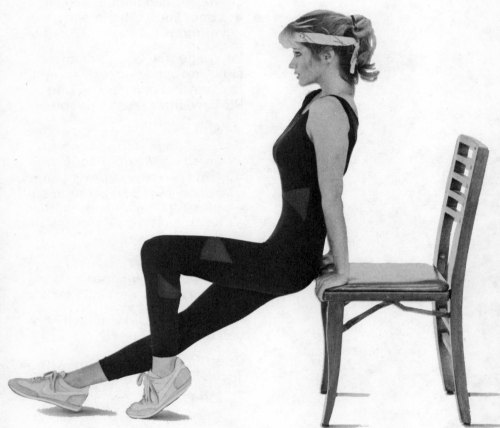

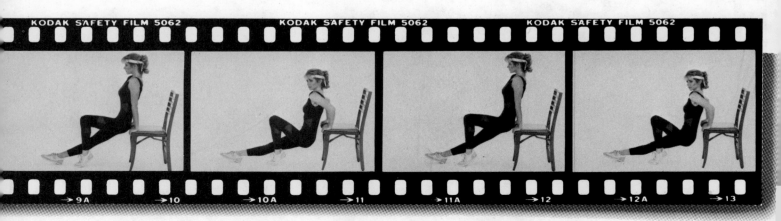

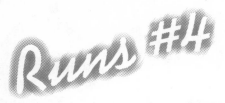

Runs #4

FOR: FOREVER!
REPS: 15x's (Both legs together is one count)
TIME: 7 seconds

This is it for the Runs. I want you to really burn it out! Down on the floor and pretend you're running for home base!

1. Support yourself on your hands and toes as though you were doing Push-ups—but with one leg extended straight out and the other flexed toward your chest. Keeping your "tushie" down, try to be STREAMLINED!

2. <u>Alternate legs</u> as if running in place, bring one knee all the way up to your chest with the other leg extended and then alternate legs and continue running while supporting yourself on your hands.

3. Each right and left together is 1 count. So, count 1, and; 2, and; up to 15 and gimme 15 in 7 seconds!

SMOKE IT!!! And keep it going right into Butt Burners or Push-ups.

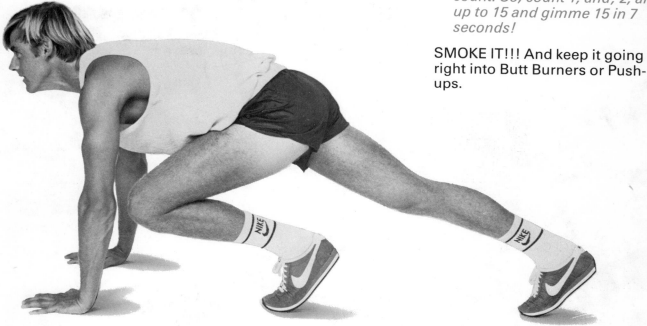

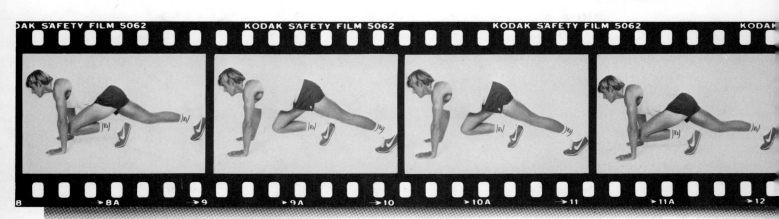

Butt Burners #4

FOR: EVERYONE ALWAYS!
REPS: 15x's each leg
TIME: 15 seconds each leg

Let's not even talk about it!

1. On hands and knees with right leg extended directly out behind you and foot pointed down.

2. Keep it tight, and raise and lower your leg trying to get it higher each time.

Feel the pressure!!
Gimme 15 on each leg *and don't quit now.*

44

Push-Ups #4

FOR: If you don't know by now look it up!
REPS: 5x's
TIME: 5 seconds

Okay, down on the floor for the last time. If these were too easy for you, great. You can add more at your next workout. But make sure you are doing the 5 Push-ups in 5 seconds...that's the truly smokin' test.

1. *Down on your hands and knees as shown.*

2. *Bending your elbows, roll forward on your knees, lower your chest towards the floor and then push yourself back to starting position. Gimme 5!*

Just keep adding those reps and maintaining your time and you'll get the killer Push-ups in the next chapter. (Maybe!)

Get ready to start to cool off!

And let's get up and go out for some Lunge!

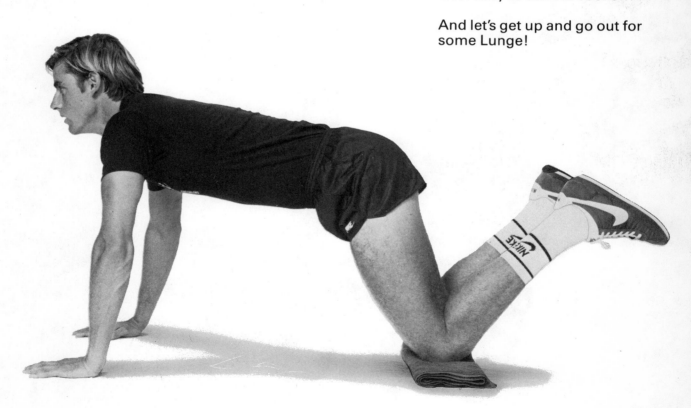

SAFETY FILM 5062

→12A   →13

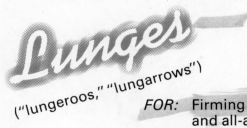

Lunges

("lungeroos," "lungarrows")

FOR: Firming thighs and buttocks and all-around flexibility

REPS: 10x's (Both legs together is one count)

TIME: 20 seconds

Okay, okay, so it's not exactly a cool off...but it's a start.

1. Stand straight with feet together and hands on hips. Keep everything nice and tight.

2. Step forward with one leg and bend the knee. Keep the other leg straight. Feel the stretch.

3. Return to standing position and repeat with the other leg.

    You got it! Gimme 10 altogether! And don't let that back leg bend...ever.

GREAT! Now I want you to get down! No, not like that...I mean get down on the floor!

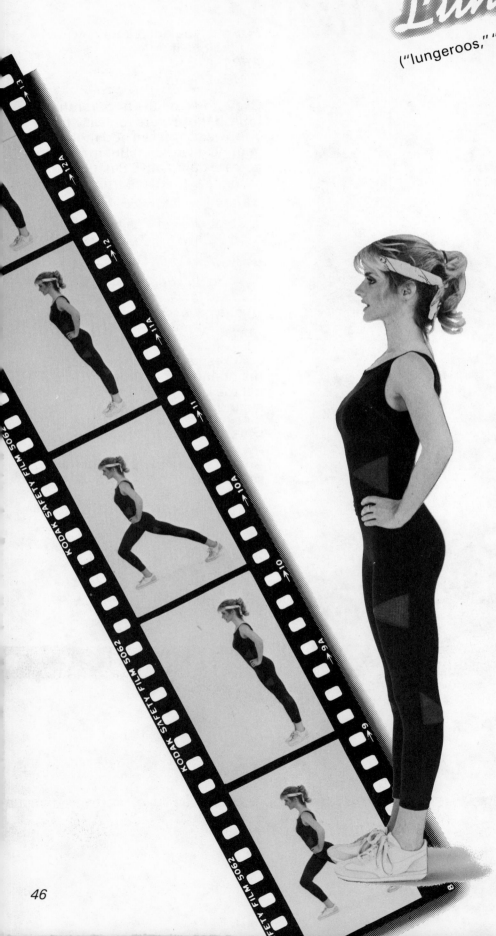

Wishbone Stretch

FOR: Stretching back of legs, middle back, lower back and inner thigh

REPS: Hold each position for 15 counts

TIME: 7 seconds each position

Enjoy this one...you're on your way home.

1. Sit on the floor with legs open in a "V" and arms held out straight in front.

2. Dropping your chin on your chest, gently reach toward toes, and return to center.

3. Repeat on the <u>left side and the right.</u>

KODAK SAFETY FILM 5062   KODAK SAFETY FILM 5062   KODAK SAFETY FILM 5062   KODAK

8   →8A   →9   →9A   →10   →10A   →11   →11A   →12

47

Hurdles
("H-U-R-T-S")

FOR: Stretching waist, hamstrings, front of legs, middle back, back of arms and lower back!

REPS: Hold for 15 counts each leg

TIME: 10 seconds each leg

Hey! You should be cooling down by now. But you gotta stretch those warmed-up and cooked muscles. You owe it to them.

1. *Still sitting in the "V" position bend one leg behind you.*

2. *Bending from the waist, slow reach for the ankle of the straight leg. Try to touch your chest (not head!) to your knee*

   Hold for count of 15.

3. *Alternate legs and repeat.*

I got one last little something for you. Would you believe I'm gonna give you an Eggroll? Hey! Trust me! This is Jake talking to you! So, go for it!

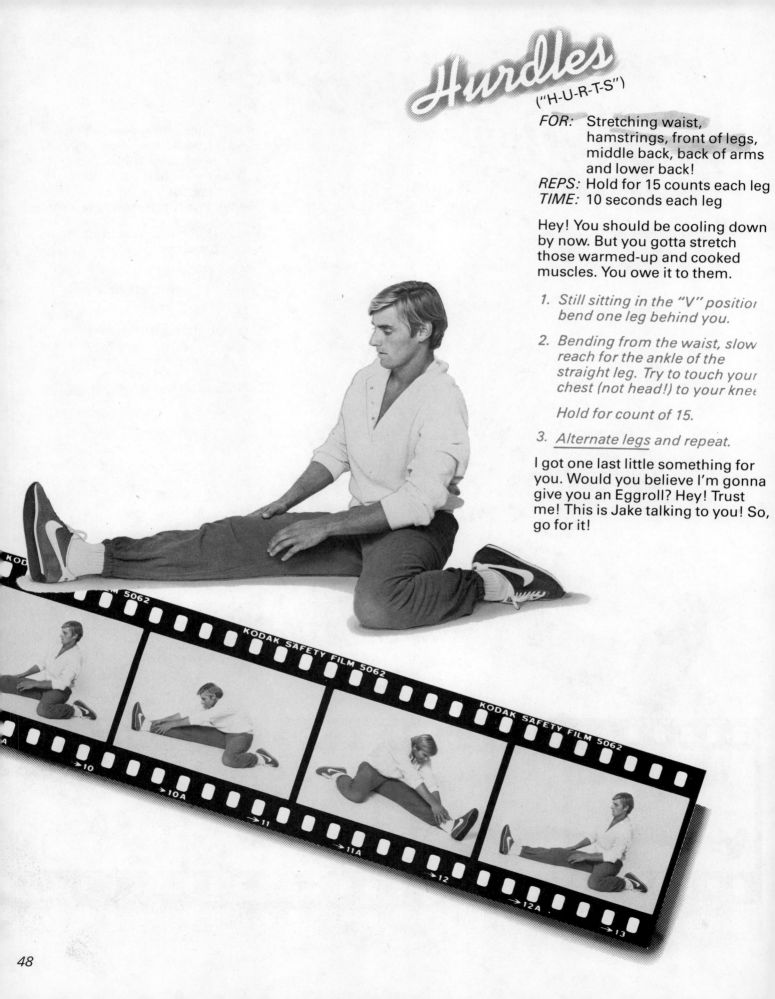

Eggroll

FOR: The final stretch to relax the spine

REPS: 1

TIME: Hold for 15 counts

This is the best Eggroll you'll ever have and I promise you that you can always have an Eggroll when you finish your workout! And Egghead: remember to put a towel or padded surface under your back, otherwise Eggroll could become "Scrambled Eggs"!

1. *Sit with knees bent and feet flat on the floor, clasp your arms around your knees and hug them to your chest.*

2. *Bring your head up as close to your knees as possible and slowly roll back vertebrae by vertebrae.*

That's it! Roll up slowly and return to standing position. Walk around! You gotta cool off!

SUPREME!!!! You did it! And I hope you did it as good as you could!

Maybe you didn't get through every exercise at top speed but that's what you've got to look forward to!

I got one last thing to say to you...so turn the page.

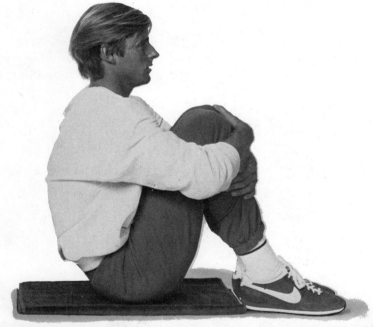

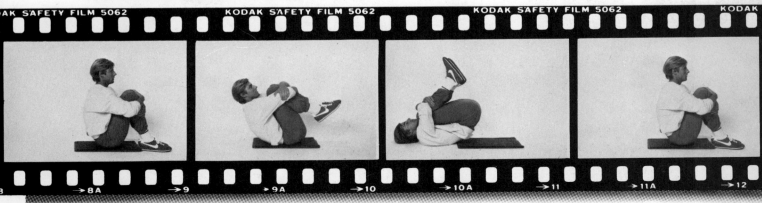

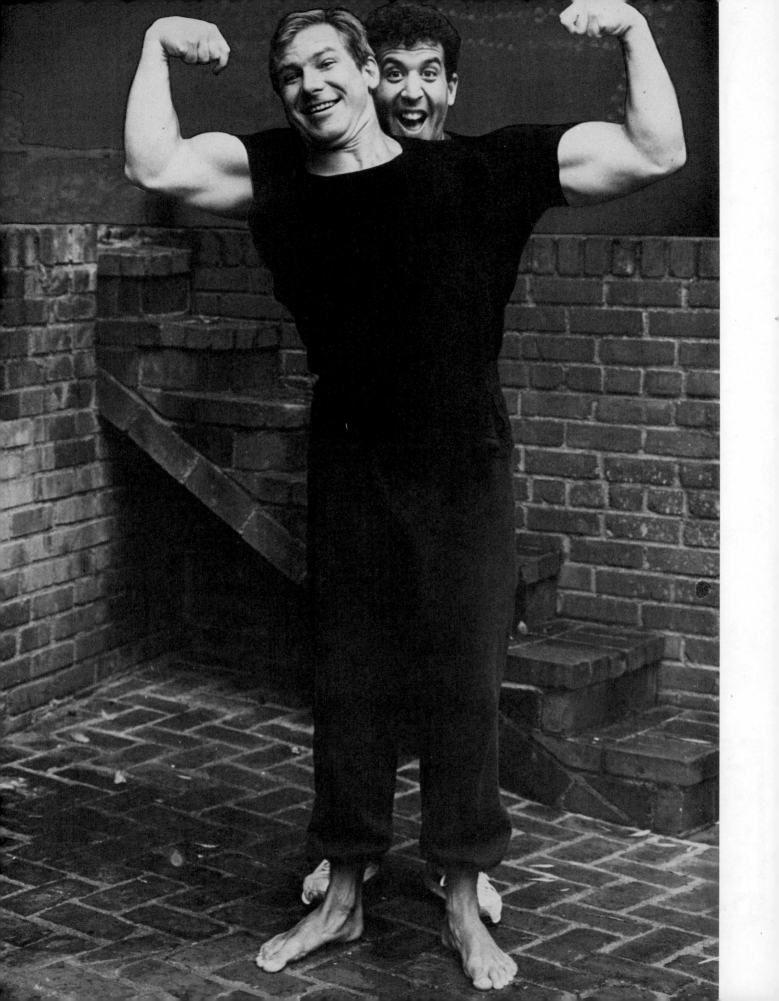

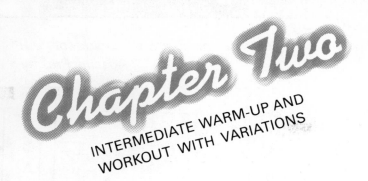

Chapter Two
INTERMEDIATE WARM-UP AND WORKOUT WITH VARIATIONS

Hey! You came back! Good job. How ya feelin'? Stronger? Ready for more? Ready to truly hustle? Bonus! But I want to talk to you for just a sec' before we go on. We need to cover a few more things.

I'm psyched that you're ready to go on to the next level. That means you got the motivation and the goal. But do you have the "info" really locked into your skull? Do you really understand my exercises? We're gonna change some of them a little bit in this chapter and if you didn't pay attention to your form in the last chapter...soreness may take on a new meaning for you. Part of learning to be physically fit is understanding the process.

So you started at the beginning and did the warm-ups EVERYTIME you did the program. Smokin'! And, now that you're not a beginner anymore you think you might skip the warm-up? Don't be a jerk! No matter what your program is, you gotta always warm-up. Warming-up, in case you hadn't noticed, is exactly that. You're raising your body's temperature from its resting level and warming-up your muscles. It's not stretching. You're trying to raise your body temp not your injury level. So always start with the BIG Stretch and...yeah I know, I said don't stretch. Well, if you look real carefully at the Big Stretch you'll see that it's really the Big Reach with no way to bounce or jerk your muscles. And get hot. Remember: you gotta exercise before you exercise!

And, the same way you can't skip any steps in the warm-up, you can't skip any steps in the workout either. I've developed this program with the reps and sets increasing gradually. So, don't fool around with a good thing! Just keep following the program charts, watch the variations and always give that last little push when you think you can't do another rep.

Look at the exercise chart and notice that some of the exercises are starred. These exercises are variations on the exercises from the last chapter. You MUST try them out BEFORE you put them in the program. I'm repeating ALL the instructions for ALL the exercises in this chapter. And we're starting the program with the same reps that we ended the last chapter with. But this is the last time I describe every exercise every time. Memorize those warm-ups and memorize those sprints...they'll never change even though you will!

INTERMEDIATE WARM-UP & WORKOUT WITH VARIATIONS
- ALL NEW EXERCISES ARE MARKED WITH A STAR
- ALL VARIATIONS ARE MARKED WITH A STAR

RECOMMEND 1 WORKOUT AT EACH LEVEL ADDING REPS AS INDICATED

CHAPTER TWO

EXERCISES	Workout 1 REPS	U DID	Workout 2 REPS	U DID	Workout 3 REPS	U DID	Workout 4 REPS	U DID	Workout 5 REPS	U DID	GOAL
BIG STRETCH	5		6		7		8		9		10
HEAD ROLLS	5		5		5		5		5		5
ARM CIRCLES	35		36		37		38		39		40
TWISTERS	35		36		37		38		39		40
* BROOMSTICK: TWISTERS	35		36		37		38		39		40
* SIDE STRETCHES	20		21		22		23		24		25
SINGLE SIDE STRETCHES	20		21		22		23		24		25
* BENT OVER TWISTERS	35		36		37		38		39		40
* SIDE: STRETCHES	10		11		12		13		14		15
SINGLES	10		11		12		13		14		15
OVER HEAD (both arms up)	10		11		12		13		14		15
SINGLE OVER HEAD	5		7		9		11		13		15
*BUTT BURNERS #1 (Women)	20		21		22		23		24		25
TOE TOUCHES	20		21		22		23		24		25
RUNS #1	20		21		22		23		24		25
PUSH-UPS #1 (Men)	10		11		12		13		14		15
RUNS #2	20		21		22		23		24		25
*INNER THIGH (Women)	20		21		22		23		24		25
PUSH-UPS #2 (Men)	10		11		12		13		14		15
*SIT-UPS	20		20		20		20		20		20/20
*LEG RAISES— IN/OUTS	20		20		20		20		20		20
SCISSORS	20		20		20		20		20		20
BABY RUNS	20		20		20		20		20		20
RUNS #3	20		21		22		23		24		25
* BUTT BURNERS #2 (Women)	20		21		22		23		24		25

EXERCISES	Workout 1 REPS	U DID	Workout 2 REPS	U DID	Workout 3 REPS	U DID	Workout 4 REPS	U DID	Workout 5 REPS	U DID	GOAL
PUSH-UPS #3 (Men)	10		10		10		10		10		10
PUSH-UPS (all)	10/20		11/21		12/22		13/23		14/24		15/25
*DOOR JAMB STRETCH	2		(HOLD FOR 15 COUNTS EACH SIDE)								2
*DOOR JAMB LATERALS	1		(HOLD FOR 10 COUNTS)				2		2		2
DOOR KNOB CURLS	15		15		15		15		15		15
*TRICEP PUSH-UPS	15		16		17		18		19		20
RUNS #4	20		21		22		23		24		25
PUSH-UPS #4	10		10		10		10		10		10
*INNER THIGH #2	20		21		22		23		24		25
*LUNGES	15		16		17		18		17		20
*WISHBONE STRETCH	1		(HOLD EACH POSITION FOR 15 COUNTS)						5		5
HURDLES	1		2		3		4		5		5

JAKE'S JARGON

barbell—bar with adjustable weights at both ends
curl—done by bending the arms at the elbow as the weight is pulled up by the bicep
dumbbell—a weight held in each hand—looks like a baby barbell
lock-out—forcing joints in the opposite direction of their normal bend
press—when a weight is lifted over head to arms length while standing, sitting or lying down.

These are the words you need to know to start with weights. I'm sure you'll have some words of your own you'll want to add *after* you've worked out.

See ya!

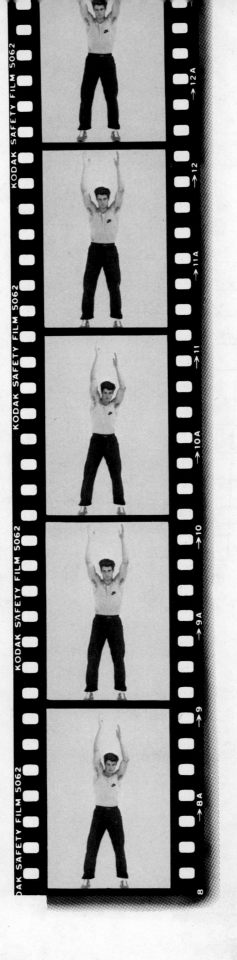

Big Stretch

FOR: Loosening up arms, middle back and waist
REPS: 5x's each side, alternating sides
TIME: 10 seconds altogether

Take this real slow and feel your body start to loosen. Then feel it get warm and then get ready to get truly HOT!

1. Stand straight, shoulders back, feet shoulder width apart and your arms raised straight up above your head with your palms facing each other.

2. _Alternately_ reach each arm in the air as far as it will go, keeping your elbows by your ears, five times for each arm.

Reach for it, "partner"! And get ready to move a little faster real soon.

Head Rolls

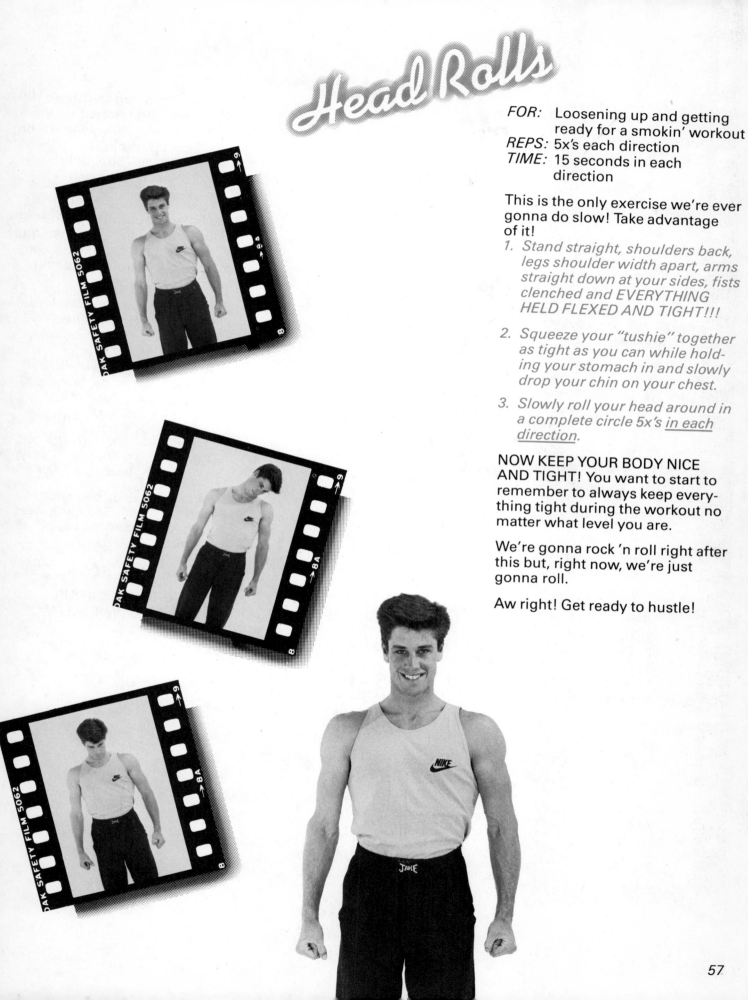

FOR: Loosening up and getting ready for a smokin' workout

REPS: 5x's each direction

TIME: 15 seconds in each direction

This is the only exercise we're ever gonna do slow! Take advantage of it!

1. *Stand straight, shoulders back, legs shoulder width apart, arms straight down at your sides, fists clenched and EVERYTHING HELD FLEXED AND TIGHT!!!*

2. *Squeeze your "tushie" together as tight as you can while holding your stomach in and slowly drop your chin on your chest.*

3. *Slowly roll your head around in a complete circle 5x's in each direction.*

NOW KEEP YOUR BODY NICE AND TIGHT! You want to start to remember to always keep everything tight during the workout no matter what level you are.

We're gonna rock 'n roll right after this but, right now, we're just gonna roll.

Aw right! Get ready to hustle!

Arm Circles

FOR: Warming up the upper body, strengthening upper back and chest, gettin' your heart pumpin'!!

REPS: 35x's each direction

TIME: 10 seconds in each direction

Okay, let's get rockin'! It's time to pick up speed and never, ever quit! You gotta get psyched! Let's light 'em up! Concentrate on keepin' everything real tight!

1. *Keep the legs shoulder width apart and bend your knees slightly. Squeeze your "tushie" real tight, flex the stomach real tight and extend your arms straight out from your shoulders as shown with fists clenched.*

2. *Swing your arms in small circles from the shoulders keeping everything nice and TIGHT!*

3. *Keep 'em rollin'! You got 10 seconds to do 35 in one direction and 10 seconds to do 35 in the opposite direction.*

   So gimme 35 in __each direction__!

FEEL IT BURN UP IN YOUR SHOULDERS! DON'T SLOW DOWN!!!

Gettin' warm? Great!

Let's get to Twisters!

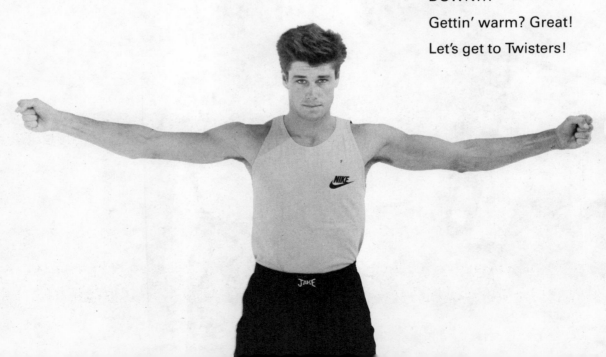

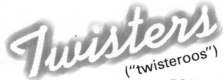

Twisters
("twisteroos")

FOR: Stretching waist, spine and upper back

REPS: 35x's (each complete twist from side to side is one count)

TIME: 10 seconds

Gotta make sure that your heart is started just in case the thought of working out with me hasn't done that already!

REMEMBER: EVERYTHING IS HELD NICE AND TIGHT!!!

1. *Stand with the knees slightly bent and the "tushie" squeezed real tight. With the arms bent in front of your chest and fists clenched, pick a point straight ahead to focus on.*

2. *Keeping head and hips in place, twist at the waist from <u>side to side</u>.*

   Gimme 35 full Twisters in ten seconds!!!!

HUSTLE!!! AND DON'T STOP!!! Keep 'em goin' now!

GREAT!!!

Get that broomstick for Twisters with a broom!

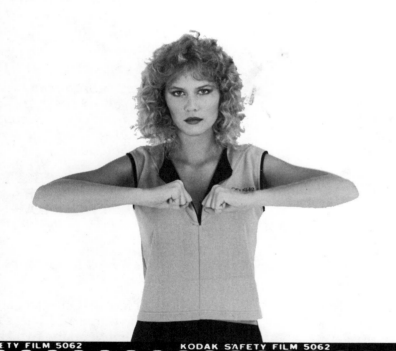

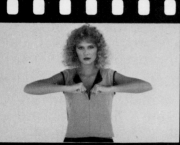
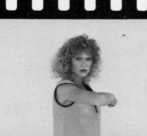
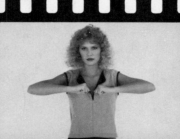
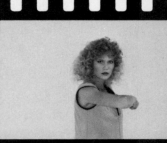

Broomstick Twisters

*

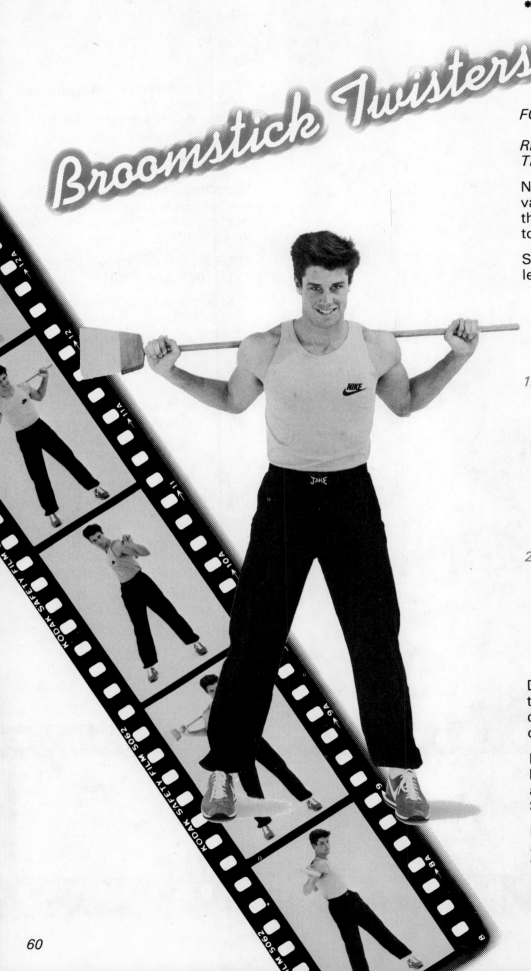

FOR: Strengthening upper body and increasing flexibility
REPS: 35x's
TIME: 12 seconds

Now, pay attention! This is the first variation. It might be harder than the old way and…it's supposed to be!

So get your broomstick in gear and let's go! AND NO SLO' MO'!!

1. *Stand with feet apart. Hold your body nice and tight with the broomstick behind you,* across the tops of your arms *instead of behind your neck.*

   Squeeze the broomstick REAL TIGHT, pick a focus point directly in front of you keeping your head and hips straight throughout the exercise.

2. *Now twist from side to side just like the other Broomstick Twister only the broomstick stays behind the tops of your arms.*

   Gimme 35 full Broomstick Twisters in 12 seconds!

Do it! You feel that stretch across the tops of your arms? That's the difference between the two kinds of Twisters.

Now, I want you to keep that broomstick across the tops of your arms for the rest of the Broomstick Stretches.

If it starts to really be uncomfortable, and I mean *REALLY* uncomfortable, then I want you to put it behind your neck but always try to increase the amount of work you do with it in this new position.

Broomstick Side Stretches ✱

FOR: Stretching rib cage and surrounding muscles

REPS: 20x's with three counts on each side—alternating sides EXAMPLE: 1,2,3; (other side) 1, 2, 3; (return to first side) 2, 2, 3; 2, 2, 3; 3, 2, 3; 3, 2, 3; etc. continuing to alternate sides

TIME: 20 seconds

IS EVERYTHING TIGHT??? Here we go! Get ready to cook!

1. Stand in same position as previous exercise.

2. Bend from <u>left to right</u> and count as above. On each stretch to the side go further—KEEP THOSE "ABBA-DABBAS" TIGHT!!!

Gimme 20 full stretches!

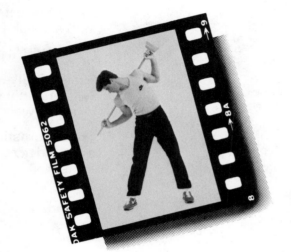

Broomstick Single Side Stretches

1. Same movement only 1 count <u>on each side</u>: 1, and; 2, and; 3, and; etc.

COME ON!!! DO IT!!! DON'T LOSE SPEED!

BONUS! You're gettin' hot!

HUSTLE!!!

61

✱ Variation from previous chapter.

Bent Over Broomstick Twisters

FOR: Stretching waist, spine, chest, shoulders, upper back, hamstrings
REPS: 35x's
TIME: 15 seconds

Okay, this is it for the broomstick stuff so LIGHT 'EM UP!

Is EVERYTHING tight??

These are like the Broomstick Twisters only you're bent over from the waist with a flat back.

The broomstick stays behind you and held across the tops of your arms.

1. Stand with feet apart, bend over from the waist keeping your knees slightly bent. Keep your back FLAT and tuck your chin into your chest.

2. Twist one way and then the other, trying to get the end of the broom to the floor on each twist down.

KEEP UP YOUR SPEED!!!

Gimme 35 full Twisters in 15 seconds.

ROCK 'EM AND GO! GO! GO!

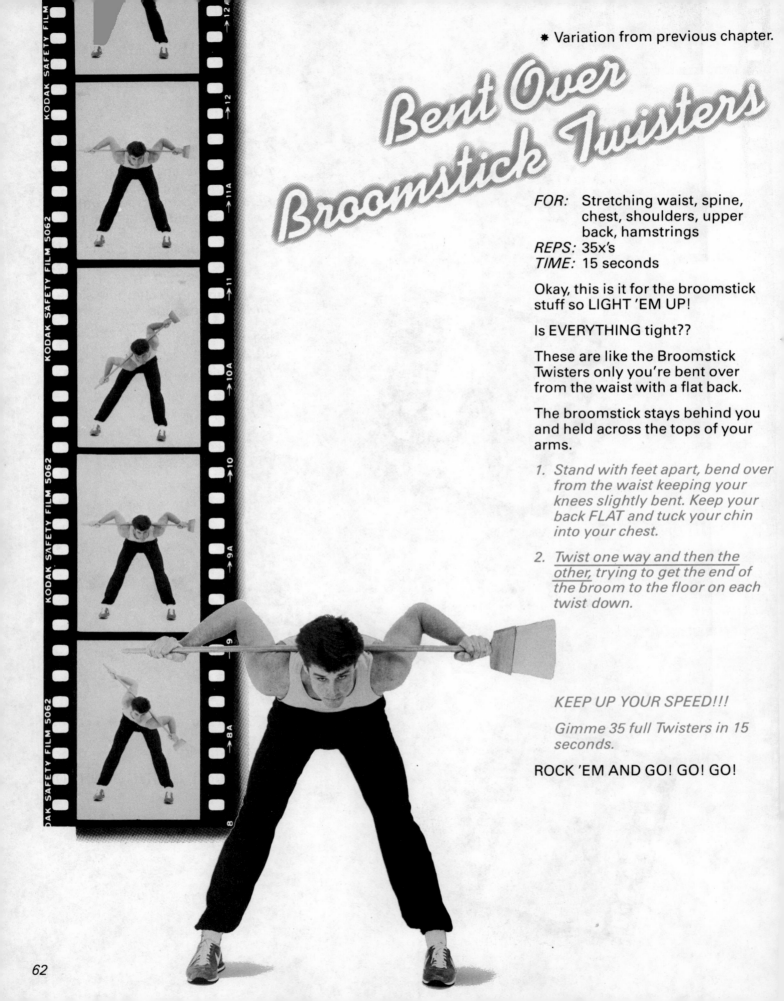

Side Stretches

FOR: Bigger stretch for the upper body

REPS: 10x's for each side for each set of stretches

TIME: 10 seconds for each set of stretches

Same set of stretches with one variation. I'm not gonna tell you where the variation is—you're just gonna have to read ALL the stretch instructions and find it yourself.

1. *Stand straight feet apart, with arms down at sides hands clenched and EVERYTHING HELD REAL TIGHT!!!*

2. *Stretch your right arm down your right leg for three FAST counts. Now the same thing on the other side. <u>Alternate sides,</u> MAINTAINING SPEED, for 10x's altogether. (COUNT: 1, 2, 3, and; 1, 2, 3, and; 2, 2, 3, and; 2, 2, 3, and; etc.)*

Single Side Stretches

1. *Keep the same body position but only 1 count on each side 10x's—1, and; 2, and; 3, and; HUSTLE!!!*

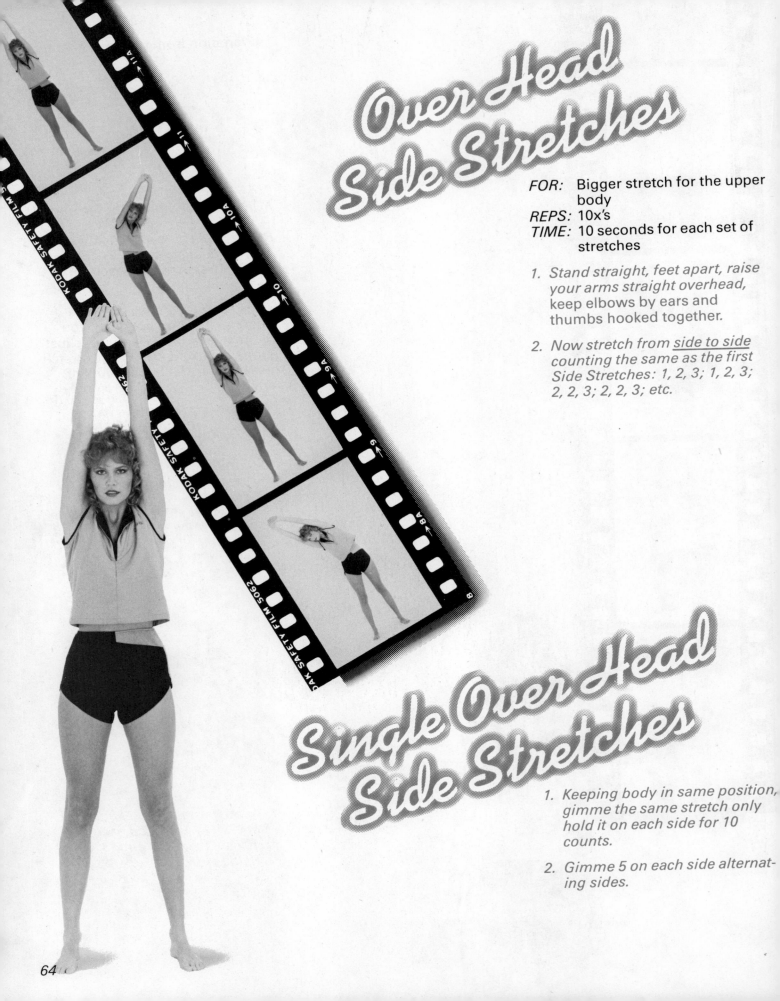

Over Head Side Stretches

FOR: Bigger stretch for the upper body
REPS: 10x's
TIME: 10 seconds for each set of stretches

1. Stand straight, feet apart, raise your arms straight overhead, keep elbows by ears and thumbs hooked together.

2. Now stretch from <u>side to side</u> counting the same as the first Side Stretches: 1, 2, 3; 1, 2, 3; 2, 2, 3; 2, 2, 3; etc.

Single Over Head Side Stretches

1. Keeping body in same position, gimme the same stretch only hold it on each side for 10 counts.

2. Gimme 5 on each side alternating sides.

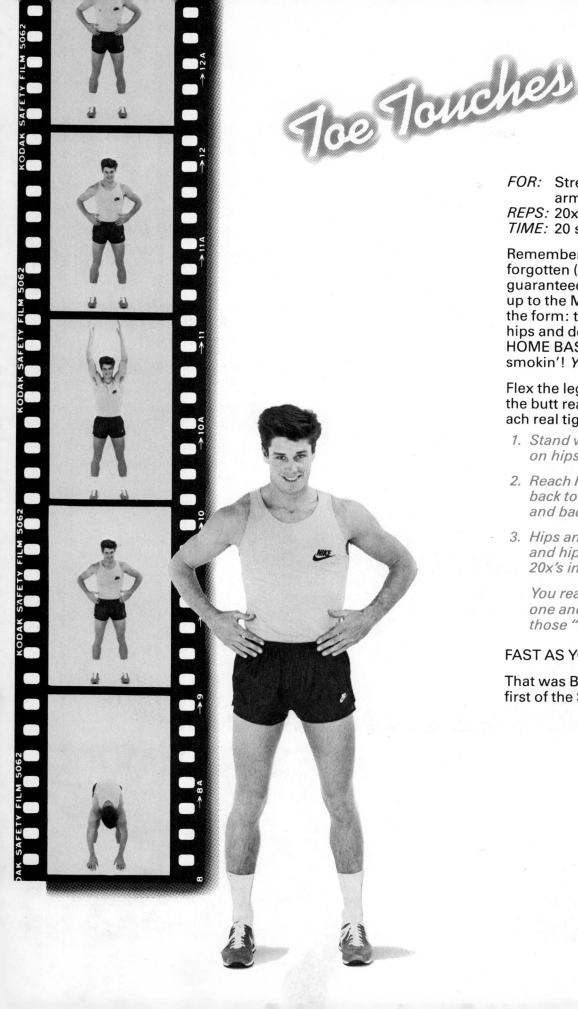

Toe Touches

FOR: Stretching hamstrings and arms
REPS: 20x's
TIME: 20 seconds

Remember these? In case you've forgotten (fat chance)...these are guaranteed to get your heart rate up to the MAX!!! Just remember the form: touch hips and up, touch hips and down. THE HIPS ARE HOME BASE! Come on, let's keep it smokin'! *You're halfway there!!!*

Flex the legs real tight! Squeeze the butt real tight! Flex the stomach real tight!

1. *Stand with feet apart and hands on hips.*

2. *Reach hands straight up, then back to hips; then down to floor and back to hips.*

3. *Hips and up and hips and down and hips and up and etc. for 20x's in 20 seconds!!!*

   You really gotta hustle on this one and feel that stretch in those "hammies."

FAST AS YOU CAN!!!

That was BONUS!!! Let's go for the first of the Steinfeld Sprints!

Runs #1

FOR: Maintaining cardio-vascular level while working arms, back, stomach, legs, calves and feet

REPS: 20x's. There are 4 sets of these spaced throughout the workout

TIME: 7 seconds

DOWN ON THE FLOOR! Lemonhead! You can't run away from them!

1. *Support yourself on your hands and toes, keeping your "tushie" down and trying to be STREAMLINED!*

2. *Alternating legs as in running, bring one knee all the way up to your chest as you straighten the opposite leg.*

3. *Count 1, and; 2, and; up to 20 and gimme 10 in 7 seconds.*

GO! GO! GO! GO! GO! GO! GO! GO! GO! GO! GO! GO! GO! GO! GO! GO!

SPRINT! SPRINT! SPRINT! SPRINT! SPRINT! SPRINT! SPRINT! SPRINT!

That's it! You got it! Keep it smokin'!

Stay down there for Butt Burners! Ladies Only!

Gentlemen! You always do Push-ups when the ladies do Butt Burners!

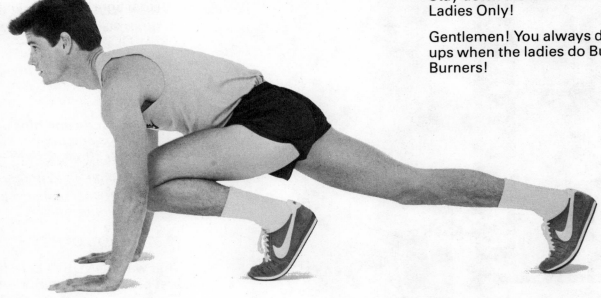

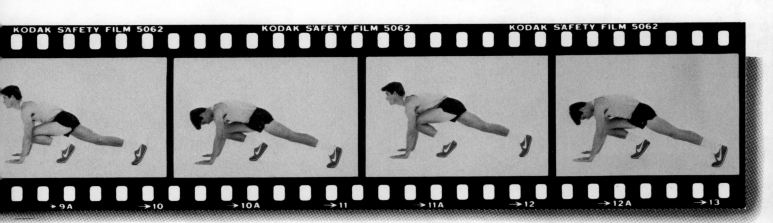

KODAK SAFETY FILM 5062   KODAK SAFETY FILM 5062   KODAK SAFETY FILM 5062

→9A   →10   →10A   →11   →11A   →12   →12A   →13

Butt Burners #1 *

FOR: GUESS!
REPS: 20x's each leg
TIME: 20 seconds each leg

There are only 2 sets of these spaced throughout the chapter and they're different than the last chapter so read them carefully!

I can't wait for you to see what replaces the other two sets!

Remember you have to use yourself as resistance in raising and lowering your leg. Just pretend I'm there exerting pressure on that leg as you try to raise it but be glad I'm not!

So let's do Butt Burners and remember to "resist yourself"... I know it's hard.

1. *On hands and knees, extend right leg directly out behind you, foot flexed AND TURNED OUT as shown. Keep your back flat!*

2. *KEEP EVERYTHING TIGHT IN CASE YOU'VE FORGOTTEN and without letting your back move, raise and lower your leg trying to get it higher each time.*

   Gimme 20 on each leg and no resting!!!

Work that leg and feel that "tushie" get smaller and smaller as it BURNS!

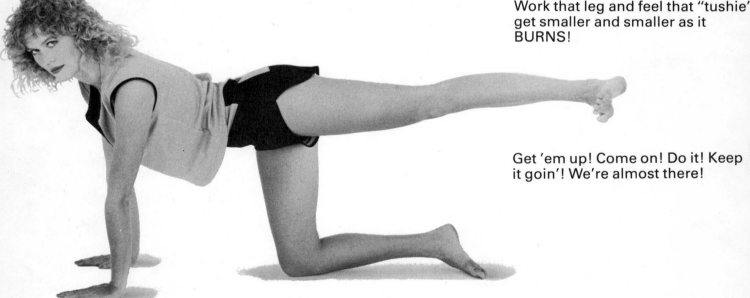

Get 'em up! Come on! Do it! Keep it goin'! We're almost there!

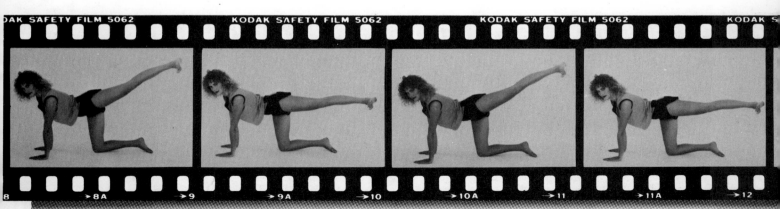

Push-Ups #1

FOR: Toning and strengthening upper body, maintaining heart rate

REPS: 10x's

TIME: 10 seconds

Don't worry. This is the last chapter with these Push-ups. We just gotta make sure that you're up to full-blown all out Push-ups before we go on.

So do your four sets of these with the additional reps for the next two weeks and Chapter Three will give you new respect for "pushers."

Now you remember how to do these...

1. *On hands and knees on floor.*

2. *Bending elbows, rolling forward on your knees LOWERING YOUR CHEST... NOT YOUR CHIN... to the floor and then pushing yourself back up to starting position.*

Keep that fanny and stomach tight and DON'T stick your "tushie" up in the air. Stay streamlined just like in the Steinfeld Sprints.

You got it. Just keep moving and gimme three more sets throughout this chapter.

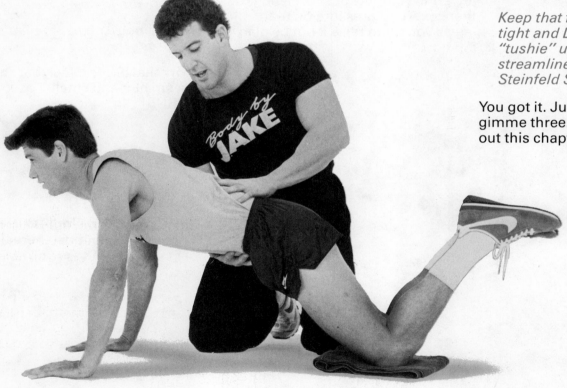

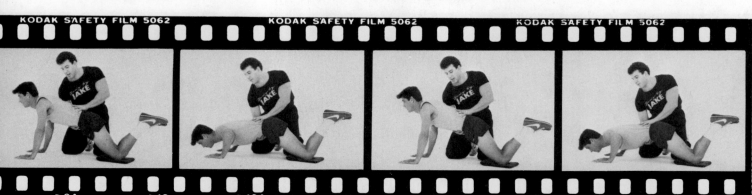

Runs #2

FOR: Maintaining cardio-vascular level! (heart rate) while working arms, back, stomach, legs, calves and feet.

REPS: 20x's (Both legs together is one count)

TIME: 7 seconds

It's your old pal…Steinfeld Sprints.

Remember to stay streamlined and stay down there until you've done them all!

Get down!

1. *Support yourself on your hands and toes as though you were doing Push-ups—but with one leg extended straight out and the other flexed toward your chest. Keeping your "tushie" down, try to be STREAMLINED!*

2. *Alternate legs as if running in place, bring one knee all the way up to your chest with the other leg extended and then alternate legs and continue running while supporting yourself on your hands.*

How'd ya do? Better? Listen, pretty soon you'll be able to do these in your sleep…as long as you sleep alone.

Let's move on…enough chit-chat. Oh, Ladies, I got something new coming up—it has to do with the inner life…the inner life of your thigh—get ready!

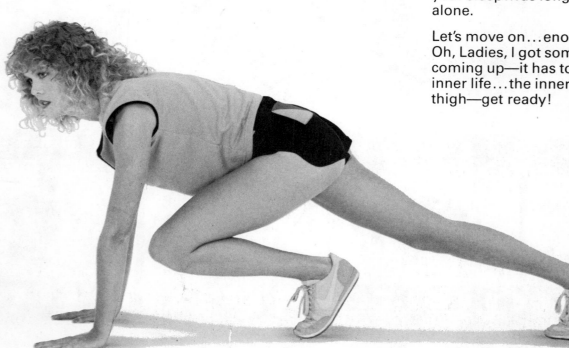

SAFETY FILM 5062 →12A →13

Inner Thigh

FOR: Firming and toning the inner thigh
REPS: 20x's each leg
TIME: 15 seconds each side

This exercise is going to work a part of your body that isn't seen all that often BUT you know they're there because you can feel them rubbing against one another! Let's put an end to that!

Down on the floor.

1. Lying on your side and supporting yourself on your elbow, bend your top knee and put your foot on the floor in front of the opposite leg and grasp the ankle.

2. Raise and lower the straight leg slowly and resist yourself just like in the Butt Burners.

3. Make sure your form is exactly like the picture otherwise you won't be able to do the variations in the next chapter. Wouldn't you hate to miss those!

So gimme 20 on <u>*each side*</u>.

Yeah, they're tough—so what? It's better than doing four sets of Butt Burners, isn't it?

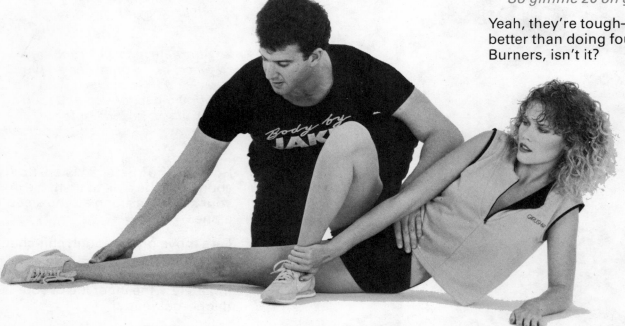

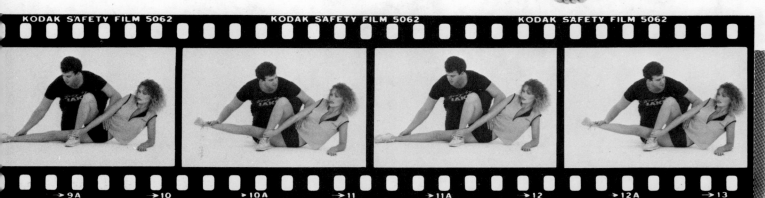

70

Push-Ups #2

FOR: Maintaining heart rate, strengthening upper body
REPS: 10x's
TIME: 10 seconds

Just be quiet and do them!

1. *On your hands and knees again.*

2. *Bending your elbows and rolling forward on your knees, lower your chest towards the floor and then push yourself back to starting position.*

Two more sets and that's it but don't forget to keep adding numbers so you can increase your stamina and speed…you're gonna need it.

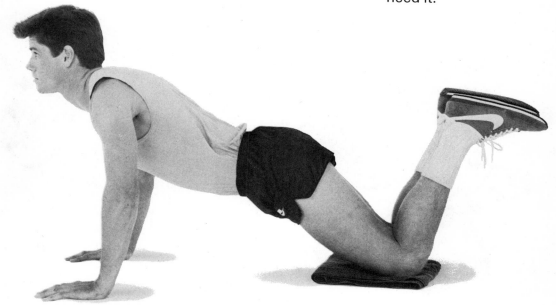

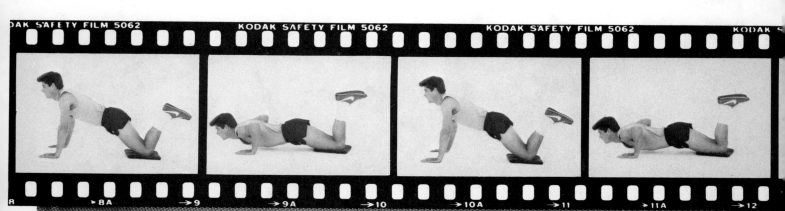

Sit-Ups*

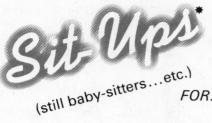

(still baby-sitters…etc.)

FOR: Waist, upper and lower "abba-dabbas" and strengthening lower back
REPS: 20x's
TIME: 20 seconds

These are sort of the same Sit-ups as the last chapter only one notch harder. (Wait 'til you get to Chapter 4!) Anyway, these have a variation that you won't find unless you read the entire instructions…

1. *Lie on the floor with your knees bent and your feet flat on the floor. CROSS YOUR ARMS OVER YOUR CHEST.*

2. *Raise your head high enough to bring your shoulder blades off the floor and then return to starting position.*

   Don't jerk yourself up!!!!!!! Gimme 20 as fast and smooth as you can while holding your stomach in.

Did you like that? You gotta remember to keep your stomach held in. Otherwise it might stick out and get stuck like that!

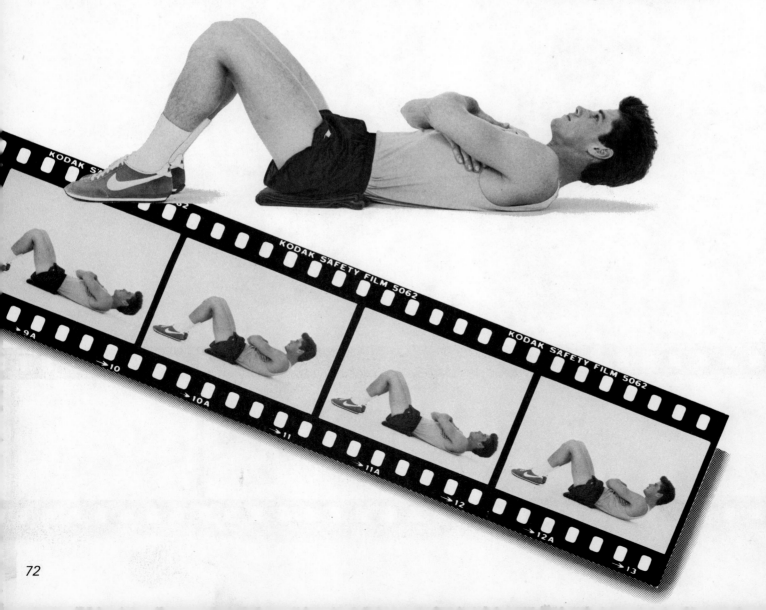

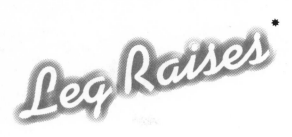

Leg Raises*

* Variation from previous chapter.

FOR: Stomach and thighs
REPS: 20x's for each set
TIME: 20 seconds for each set

These three exercises must be done together! And, you can't stop in between! Got me? We're gonna do In/Outs, Scissors, and Baby Runs. How are these different than the old Leg Raises??? Read on...

In/Outs

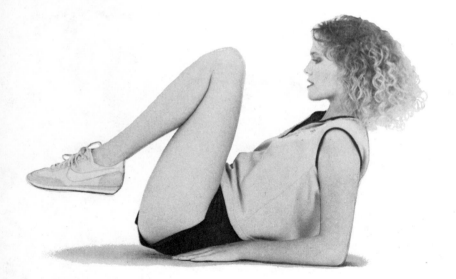

1. Lie on your back PROPPED UP ON YOUR ELBOWS (aha!) here we go.

2. Bring your knees in to your chest then push them straight out again.

3. Repeat by pulling knees up to chest again and pushing out.

Gimme a smokin' 20 and go on to Scissors. Don't let your feet touch the floor during or between the exercises!

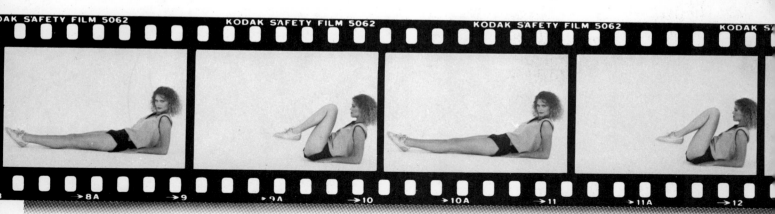

Scissors

1. Next 20: Start in same position with legs extended straight out parallel to the floor and held tight.

2. Criss-cross your legs back and forth for 20 and, GET TOUGH!

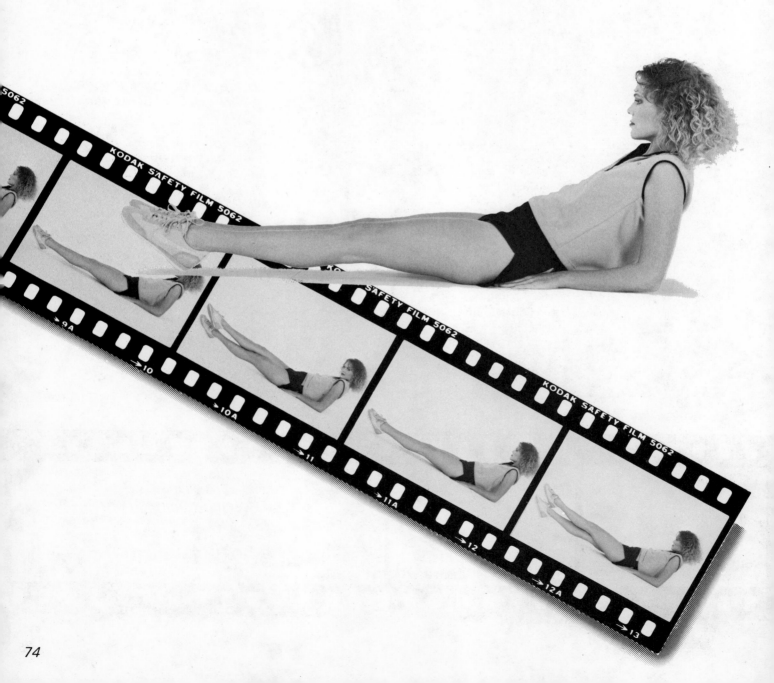

Baby Runs

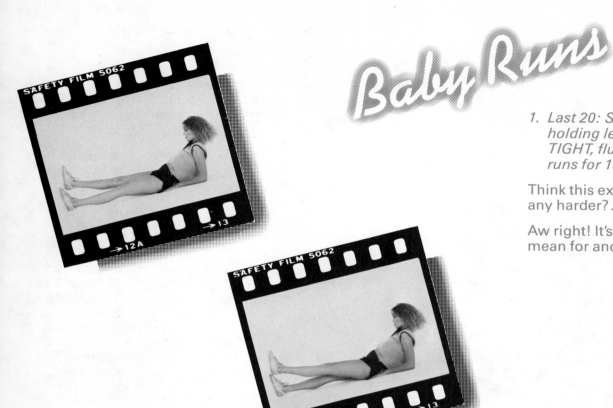

1. Last 20: Start in same position, holding legs straight and TIGHT, flutter stiff legs in tiny runs for 15 counts.

Think this exercise couldn't get any harder?...wait and see!

Aw right! It's time to get lean and mean for another 20 runs!

Runs #3*

**Variation from previous chapter.

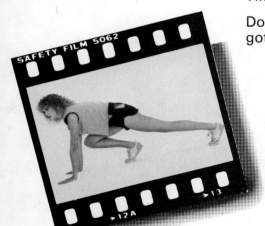

FOR: Maintaining cardio-vascular level while working arms, back, stomach, legs, calves and feet

REPS: 20x's. This is the third set of 4

TIME: 7 seconds

Do you know what to do??? You gotta GET DOWN!

1. *Support yourself on your hands and toes as though you were doing Push-ups—but with one leg extended straight out and the other flexed toward your chest. Keeping your "tushie" down, try to be STREAMLINED!*

2. *Alternate legs as if running in place, bring one knee all the way up to your chest with the other leg extended and then alternate legs and continue running while supporting yourself on your hands.*

GO FOR IT!!!

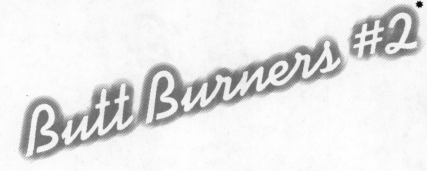

Butt Burners #2 *

FOR: "Tushies" around the world
REPS: 20x's each leg.
TIME: 20 seconds each leg

This is your next to the last time to try and work your butt off! Literally...

1. *On hands and knees as shown, extend right leg directly out behind you with foot pointed down.*

   KEEP EVERYTHING TIGHT IN CASE YOU'VE FORGOTTEN!

2. *Raise and lower your leg trying to get it higher each time. Feel the pressure and gimme 20 on* each leg *and NO RESTING!!!*

Let's do some work on that upper body, madam!

KEEP EVERYTHING TIGHT!

2. *Raise and lower your leg trying to get it higher each time. Feel the pressure and gimme 20 on each leg and NO RESTING!!!*

Now let's do some work on that upper body, madam!

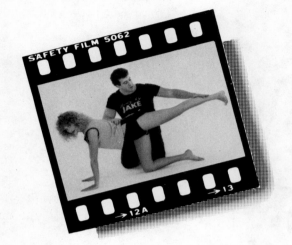

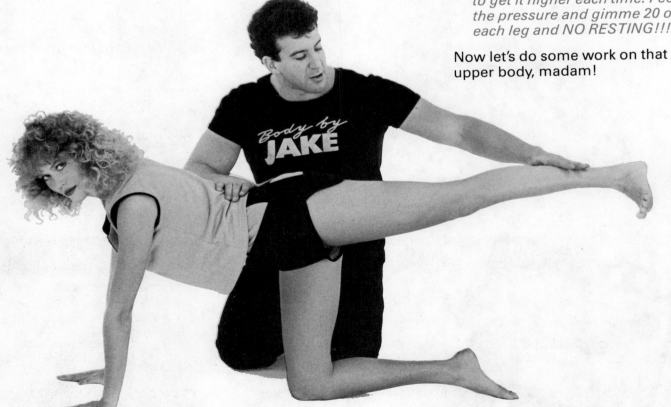

Push-Ups #3

FOR: Keepin' it cookin'
REPS: 10x's
TIME: 10 seconds

Yeah, yeah, I know but just do 'em and let's light 'em up!

1. *On your hands and knees as before.*

2. *Bending your elbows and rolling forward on your knees, lower your chest towards the floor and then push yourself back to starting position.*

3. *Do these fast, fast, fast and hold that stomach and fanny tight, tight, tight.*

I'll make them more interesting just as soon as I think you can stand the excitement.

Let's keep hustling and do some upper body work and then... we're through!

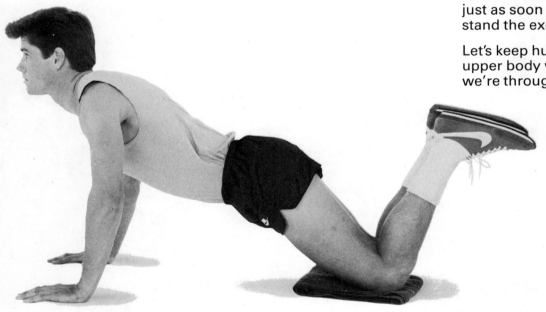

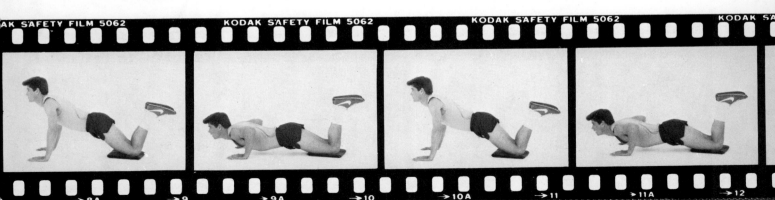

Push-Ups

FOR: Upper body and main-
taining heart rate
REPS: Ladies: 10x's Men: 20x's
TIME: 10 seconds/20 seconds

All right fellas! I know you just did Push-ups but I want you to do another set with the ladies… I'm sure it couldn't hurt!

These are the same Push-ups we've been doing with more numbers.

1. *On hands and knees.*

2. *Rolling forward on knees, bend-ing elbows and keeping fanny tucked under, lower chest to the floor (NOT YOUR CHIN).*

3. *Using arms, push yourself back up to starting position.*

I wanna remind you to keep your "tushie" tucked under. It makes me ache all over when I see someone doing Push-ups with their fanny sticking up in the air…

Now, go find a door but don't leave!

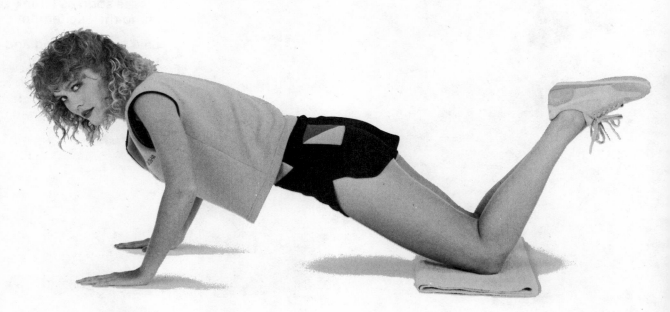

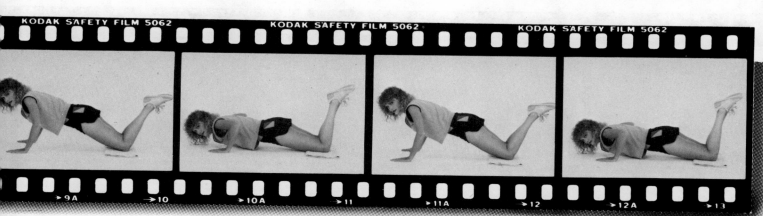

Door Jamb Stretch

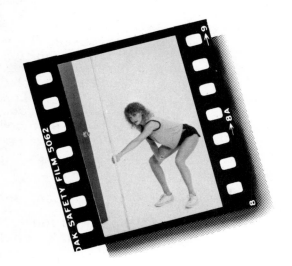

FOR: Stretching out
REPS: Hold for 15 counts on each side—TWICE
TIME: 30 seconds

This is sort of like the last Door Jamb Stretch only different. Get the picture. You gotta read the instructions.

1. *Stand grasping the door jamb as shown with only one arm at a time.*

2. *Slowly sit back on your heels and feel the stretch from the top of your side all the way down into your waist. Hold.*

3. *Now reverse and grip the door jamb the opposite way.*

   Keep reversing sides until you have done two <u>on each side</u>.

Make sure you always do the same amount of stretches on each side. Otherwise you might end up with one arm longer than the other...

Anyway, let's go on because I got another new one for you.

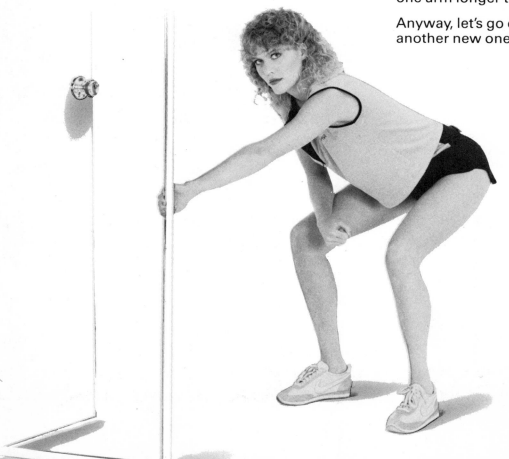

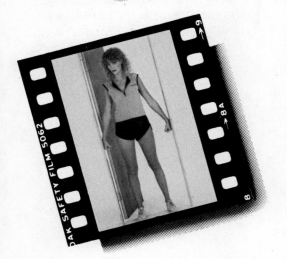

Door Jamb Laterals*

* New exercise.

FOR: Maintaining heart rate and strengthening shoulders
REPS: Hold for 10 seconds ONCE
TIME: 10 seconds

This is a good exercise to do to get you ready for some weights. It's also a good way to relieve tension.

Read Carefully.

1. *Stand in doorway with arms at sides, clenching fists. Slowly open your arms until they touch the door jamb.*

2. *Now continue to press against the door jamb for 10 seconds.*

How'd you do? Did the house fall down? It didn't!? Then ya gotta do it harder next time!

Okay, grab the door knob and get ready for some Door Knob Curls.

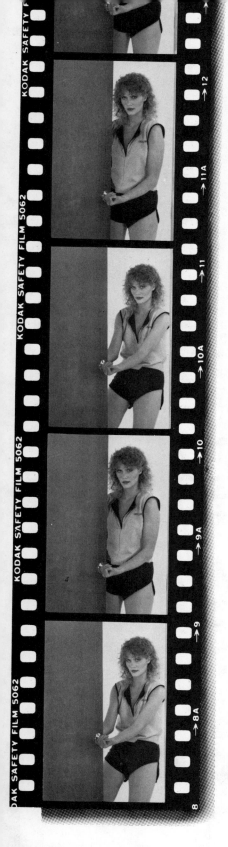

Door Knob Bicep Curls *

FOR: Guess!
REPS: 15x's
TIME: 30 seconds

Notice the time for these. I want you to really resist coming up. I want the sweat to run down your arms so you can barely hold on to the door knob. I want you to feel like your biceps are going to burst through your skin.

What do you mean, "who cares what you want???!!!".

1. *Stand facing the edge of the door, grasping the door knobs on either side of the door.*

2. *Sitting back on your heels, slowly pull yourself back towards the door using your upper arm and NOT your back to pull yourself up to starting position.*

3. *Slowly lower yourself back to sitting position and continue as directed for 15 times.*

So what if these are boring! Don't you realize that in the next chapter you get to use real live weights to do them and by doing this exercise you won't hurt yourself on the real thing!

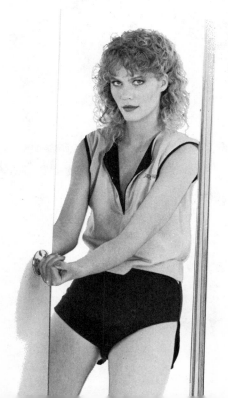

Tricep Push-Ups *

("trimens")

FOR: Backs of upper arms
REPS: 15x's
TIME: 15 seconds

Stick in there, you're really doing a good job no matter what I say and what you think.

These have a itsy-bitsy, teeny-weeny variation....

1. Sit on edge of seat, extend BOTH legs in front of you, grip the bench and raise your "tushie" off the seat.

2. Lower yourself toward the floor keeping your elbows close to your body. Raise up to starting position.

Gimme 15!

These are suddenly a little harder now, aren't they? Think two weeks with this chapter will be long enough for ya?!

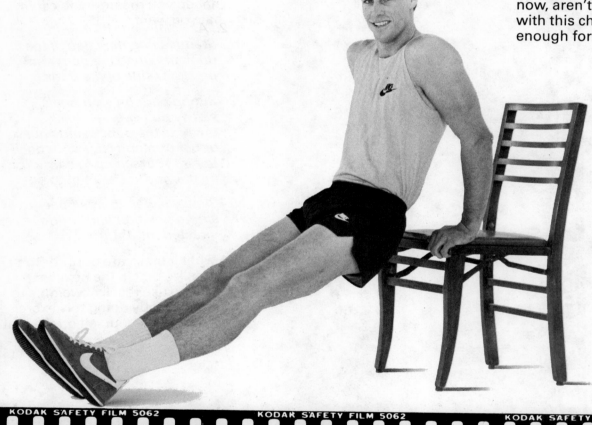

KODAK SAFETY FILM 5062   KODAK SAFETY FILM 5062   KODAK SAFETY FILM 5062

→9A   →10   →10A   →11   →11A   →12   →12A   →13

Runs #4

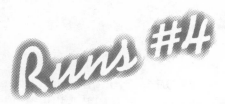

FOR: Maintaining heart rate
while working arms, back,
stomach, legs, calves, feet
and mouth (you gotta
be screaming for mercy
by now!)
REPS: 20x's
TIME: 7 seconds

This is the last time I'm gonna explain Runs. (They're ALWAYS a part of the program and they NEVER change.)

So let's get down and…get goin'!

1. *Support yourself on your hands and toes as though you were doing Push-ups—but with one leg extended straight out and the other flexed toward your chest. Keeping your "tushie" down, try to be STREAMLINED!*

2. *Alternate legs as if running in place, bring extended knee all the way up to your chest as you extend other leg and continue running while supporting yourself on your hands.*

After all this, I truly hope that the next time you see "RUNS" in the program you'll fall right down on the floor and know what to do!

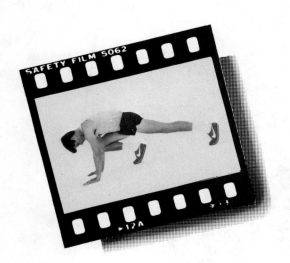

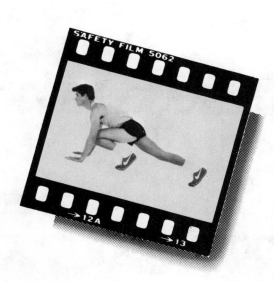

Push-Ups #4

FOR: Strengthening upper body and maintaining heart rate
REPS: 10x's
TIME: 10 seconds

All right! All right! You don't have to read the instructions. Just go ahead. But for all you conscientious exercisers I shall include them nonetheless.

1. *On hands and knees.*

2. *Bending elbows and rolling forward on knees, lower your CHEST to the floor.*

3. *Return to starting position by pushing yourself up with your arms.*

Thank you very much.

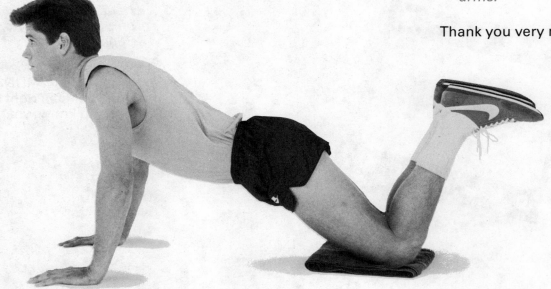

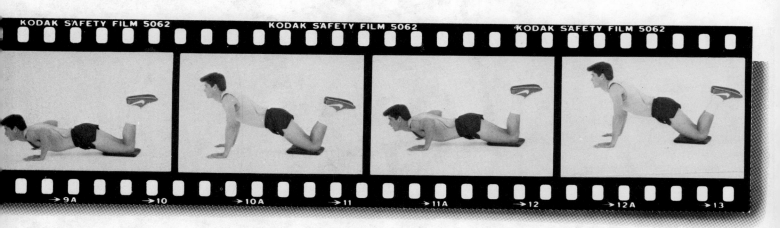

KODAK SAFETY FILM 5062   KODAK SAFETY FILM 5062   KODAK SAFETY FILM 5062

→9A   →10   →10A   →11   →11A   →12   →12A   →13

Inner Thigh #2

FOR: Firming and toning inner thigh

REPS: 20x's each side

TIME: 15 seconds each leg

I know you did these once but ya gotta do 'em twice in each workout.

Like I said, just make sure your form is "on the money" because these will always be a part of the program.

All right ladies, down on the floor.

1. Lying on your side and supporting yourself on your elbow, bend your top knee and put your foot on the floor in front of the opposite leg and grasp the ankle.

2. Raise and lower the straight leg slowly and resist yourself just like in the Butt Burners. Gimme 20 smokin' reps.

Almost through! So get the broomstick for a little surprise.

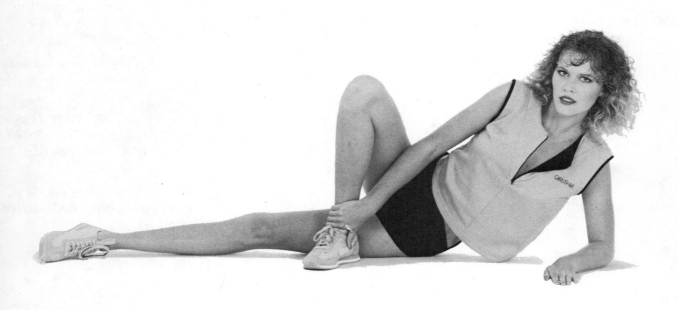

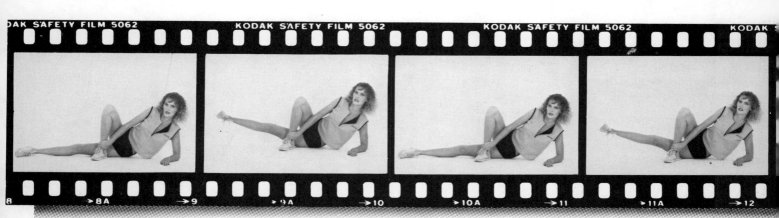

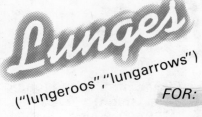

Lunges

("lungeroos","lungarrows")

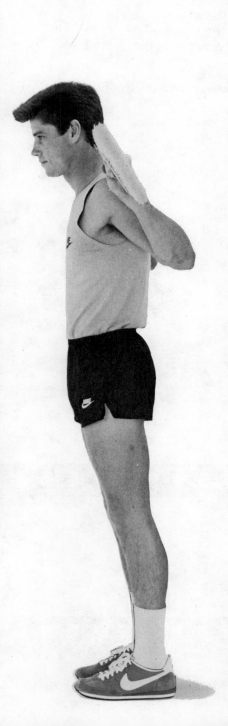

FOR: Strengthening back and firming buttocks and upper leg

REPS: 15x's (both legs together is 1 count)

TIME: 20 seconds

These are special Lunges with a BROOMSTICK! So get the broomstick and let's go out for some lunge.

1. *Stand straight with the broomstick behind neck and hands squeezing stick.*

2. *Step forward as far as you can on your left foot and bend your knee keeping the right leg extended straight behind you.*

3. *Return to starting position and alternate legs.*

HOLD YOUR HEAD AND TORSO STRAIGHT THROUGHOUT THIS EXERCISE AND DON'T LET THAT BACK LEG DROOP NEAR THE FLOOR!!!!

The broomstick made it a little more interesting huh? Did you lose your balance?

Well, that's it so get on the floor and we'll stretch it out!

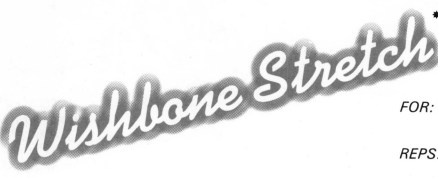

Wishbone Stretch *

FOR: Stretching back of legs, middle back, lower back and inner thigh

REPS: Hold each position for 15 counts

TIME: 7 seconds each position

This oughta feel real good after what you've gone through! Just to keep you on your toes it's a little bit different...

1. *Sit on the floor with legs open wide dropping your chin to your chest and raising your arms so your inner elbow is by your ear.*

2. *Slowly drop your body forward WITHOUT reaching.*

3. *Return to starting position and do the same thing for <u>both left and right sides</u>. DON'T BOUNCE AND DON'T FORCE A STRETCH!*

We've got one last stretch and you are THROUGH!!! For today.

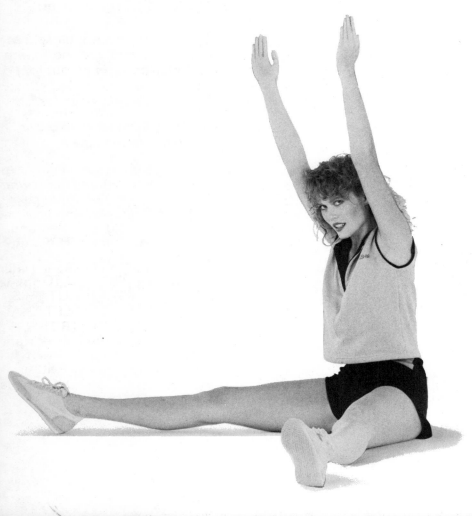

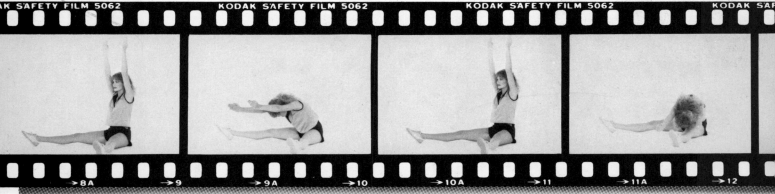

Hurdles
("H-U-R-T-S")

FOR: Stretching waist, hamstrings, front of legs, middle back, back of arms and lower back! Did I miss anything?

REPS: Hold for 15 counts each leg

TIME: 10 seconds each leg

This is it! Relax and recover!

1. Sit with legs spread wide. Bend one leg behind you, extending other leg straight out in front of you and arms extended above head with elbows by ears.

2. Bending from waist, slowly reach for your ankle.

3. While trying to touch your chest to your knee, hold for 15 counts

   Now the other leg.

BONUS!!! You did it. Is it getting easier? Do you feel any different?

Sometimes getting in shape is discouraging but just remember how long it took you to get out of shape!

There's also something important have to tell you so while you're cooling down…read on.

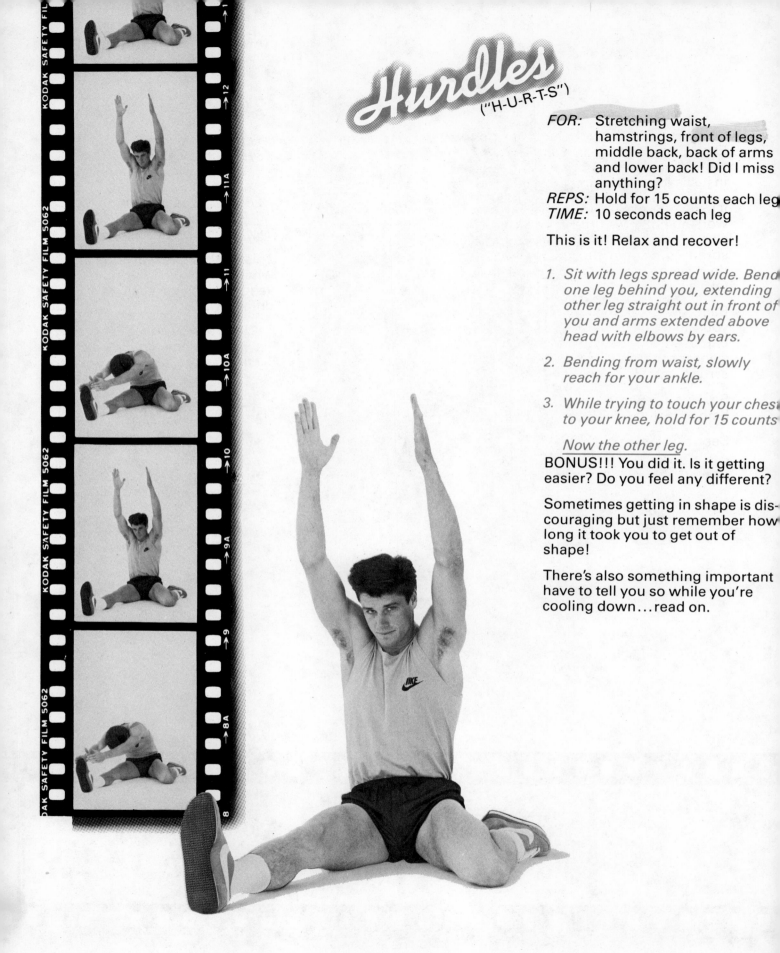

Soreness! Did you have any in the last chapter? I'm sure you did. Don't worry about it. Everybody and I mean every "body" gets sore when they first start training. It's not a bad thing. It just means you're using muscles in a way you haven't used them before...or maybe in just a long time. So, everytime you vary an exercise you're gonna get sore all over again.

It usually takes 12 to 48 hours for soreness to develop. And, it *will* go away. Since you're working out three times a week, you got a couple of days rest in between workouts and that should take care of it. If it doesn't, and the soreness feels like more than simple muscle soreness...get to the doctor. Otherwise, don't quit. Just exercise at a slower pace and maybe don't go on to the next level until the soreness goes away. And be good to yourself. Maybe take a bath!

Baths are great and will make you feel a whole lot better. Put some herbs or minerals in and you can relax and revitalize your whole system. And, remember these three things about baths: a warm bath will relax and relieve tensions, a hot bath will make you sweat which cleanses the skin, eases sore muscles and invigorates you and a cold bath will make you scream real loud.

So, if you get sore from your workout—don't get sore with Jake here! Just relax, maybe take a bath and always be good to yourself. You've worked real hard and you deserve it!

See ya in a couple of days.

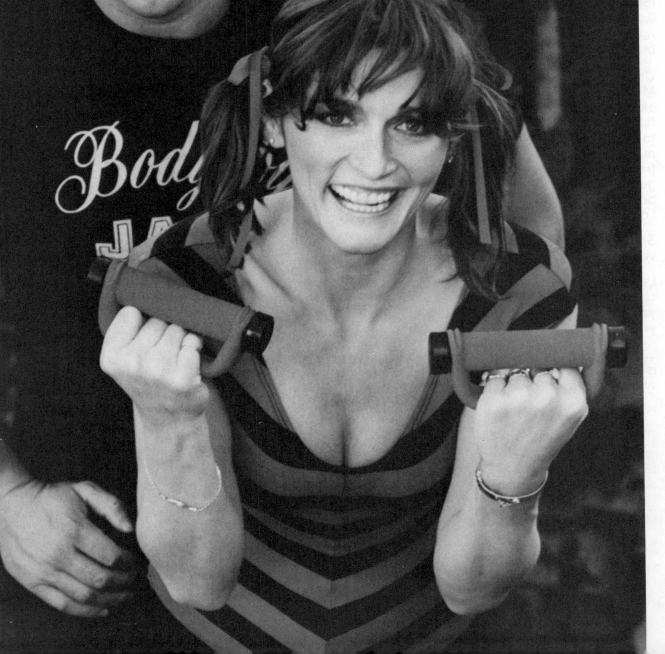

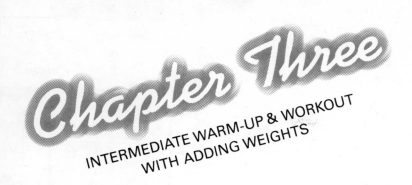

Chapter Three

INTERMEDIATE WARM-UP & WORKOUT WITH ADDING WEIGHTS

Well, it's been a month now. You feelin' good? I hope so because we're getting into some real heavy stuff now. Weights! First of all, I don't want weights to scare you! Everyone always thinks of weights and musclemen and that's not the way it is. Weights can make your body look anyway you want it to. If you want to develop size and strength then you need to train with heavy weights doing fewer repetitions. If you want to tone and trim your body then you need to use moderate weights with more repetitions. If you want to maintain your skinny, under-developed saggy shape then don't use any weights at all!

Using weights doesn't necessarily mean you'll lose pounds while you're toning your muscles. Muscle weighs three times more than fat! So even though you may be dieting and literally exercising your "tushie" off, your actual weight may be staying the same. And, you can't turn fat into muscle. I don't know who thought that up but, it's not true! Fat is fat and muscle is muscle. Fat cells will shrink when the fat is used as energy but, you always keep the same number of fat cells. Muscle does burn more calories per pound than fat though. So, by training with weights you: get more lean muscle tissue which burns more calories, thereby getting rid of unsightly fat and toning your body, leading to improved mental attitude, and possibly improving your productivity. Sounds like training with weights can change your life? I don't know why not—changed mine!

So let's get rockin' and rollin'. There is some additional equipment you'll need, some new vocabulary and some new rules and regulations concerning weight training.

Let's talk about the equipment. First of all, weights are still optional in this chapter. The next chapter you really will benefit by using weights, but in this chapter I've given you alternates if you don't want to start with the weights right now. Even if you aren't using weights now, you'll still need to know the rest of this stuff. So, here goes.

Ladies, I want you to start with a pair of 2-3 lb. dumbbells. I suggest the kind where the weight is built in and not held in place by bolts and screws. It's too easy to have these slip off during a workout and you probably won't ever want more weight anyway!

Gentlemen, I would like you to start with 10 lb. dumbbells. If you should choose to also buy barbells for presses, get an experienced salesman to help you and tell him Jake sent you.

So, get yourself psyched! Get ready for something new! And hustle! You should be real familiar with the first half of this program by now so light em' up and try and do all the reps suggested. By the time you get to the weights you should be smokin'!!!!

You're starting to be on your own now but I think you've got the information and, one would hope, some of the skills to take care of yourself! So, get mean and lean!

One last thing, don't "lock out". When you lift the weight to the top of the position and when you return to the starting position, STOP before you're fully extended and the joint is locked. I'll tell you "why" later on after you've tested the exercises.

91

INTERMEDIATE WARMUP & WORKOUT WITH THE ADDITION OF WEIGHTS

- READ EACH EXERCISE CAREFULLY   • TRY SLOWLY
- ONLY THEN PROCEED WITH COMPLETE PROGRAM
- WOMEN USE 2-3 LBS.   • MEN USE 10 LBS.

CHAPTER THREE

EXERCISES	Workout 1 REPS	Workout 1 U DID	Workout 2 REPS	Workout 2 U DID	Workout 3 REPS	Workout 3 U DID	Workout 4 REPS	Workout 4 U DID	Workout 5 REPS	Workout 5 U DID	GOAL
BIG STRETCH	10										10
HEAD ROLLS	5										5
ARM CIRCLES	40				45						50
TWISTERS	40				45						50
* BROOMSTICK: TWISTERS	40				45						50
SIDE STRETCHES	25				30						30
SINGLE SIDE STRETCHES	25				30						30
BENT OVER TWISTERS	40				45						50
* SIDE: STRETCHES	15				20						20
SINGLES	15				20						20
OVER HEAD	15				20						20
SINGLE OVER HEAD	15				20						20
TOE TOUCHES	25				30						35
RUN #1	25				30						30
*ADVANCED BUTT BURNERS #1	25				25						25
* PUSH-UP #1 (Men)	5				7						10
RUNS #2	25				30						30
*ADVANCED INNER THIGH #1 (Women)	25				25						25
PUSH-UPS #2 (Men)	5				7						10
COMBO SITTERS	20/20				25/25						30/30
*ADVANCED LEG RAISES IN/OUT	20				25						30
SCISSORS	20				25						30
BABY RUNS	20				25						30
RUNS #3	25				30						30

EXERCISES	Workout 1 REPS	Workout 1 U DID	Workout 2 REPS	Workout 2 U DID	Workout 3 REPS	Workout 3 U DID	Workout 4 REPS	Workout 4 U DID	Workout 5 REPS	Workout 5 U DID	GOAL
ADVANCED BUTT BURNERS #2	25				25						25
PUSH-UPS #3 (Men)	5				7						10
PUSH-UPS (all)	15/25				15/25						15/25
DOOR JAMB STRETCH	15				15						15
DUMBBELL PRESSES or	10				11						12
ARM CIRCLES	50				50						50
*BICEP CURL or	10				11						12
DOOR KNOB CURL	20				20						20
TRICEP PUSH-UP	10				11						12
RUNS #4 (Men)	25				30						30
ADVANCED INNER THIGH #2	25				25						25
PUSH-UPS #4 (Men)	5				7						10
*BROOMSTICK LUNGES	20				20						20
HURDLES	15		(HOLD FOR 20 COUNTS EACH POSITION)								25
WISHBONE STRETCH	15		(HOLD FOR 15 COUNTS EACH POSITION)								25

Big Stretch

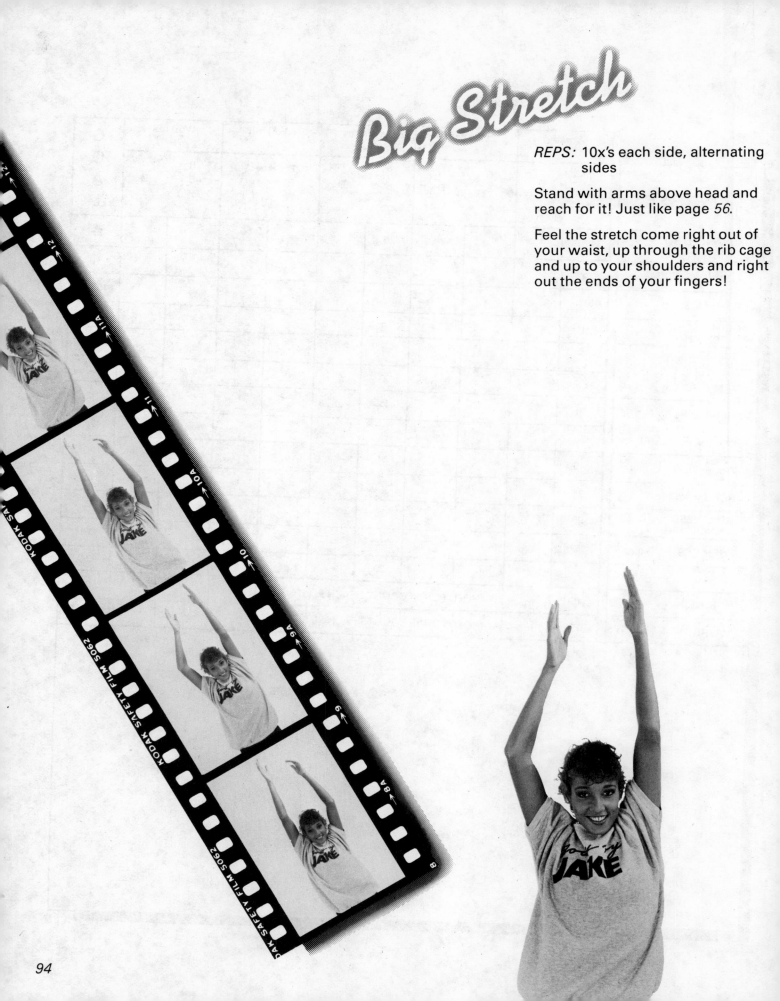

REPS: 10x's each side, alternating sides

Stand with arms above head and reach for it! Just like page *56.*

Feel the stretch come right out of your waist, up through the rib cage and up to your shoulders and right out the ends of your fingers!

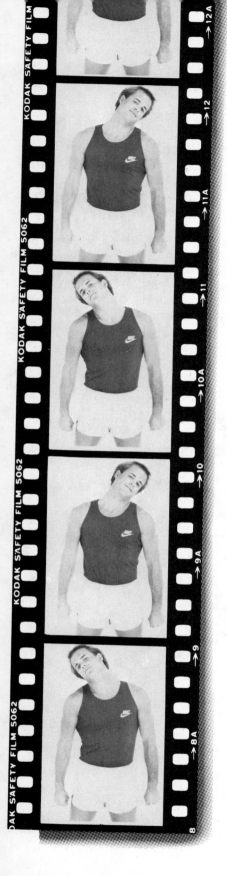

Head Rolls

REPS: 5x's each direction

Stand with arms at sides, everything held tight and gently roll your head in full circles 5 times in each direction. If you've forgotten, roll your eyes back to page 57.

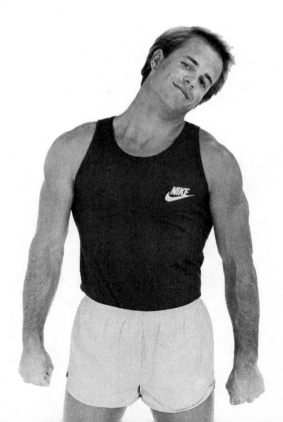

Arm Circles

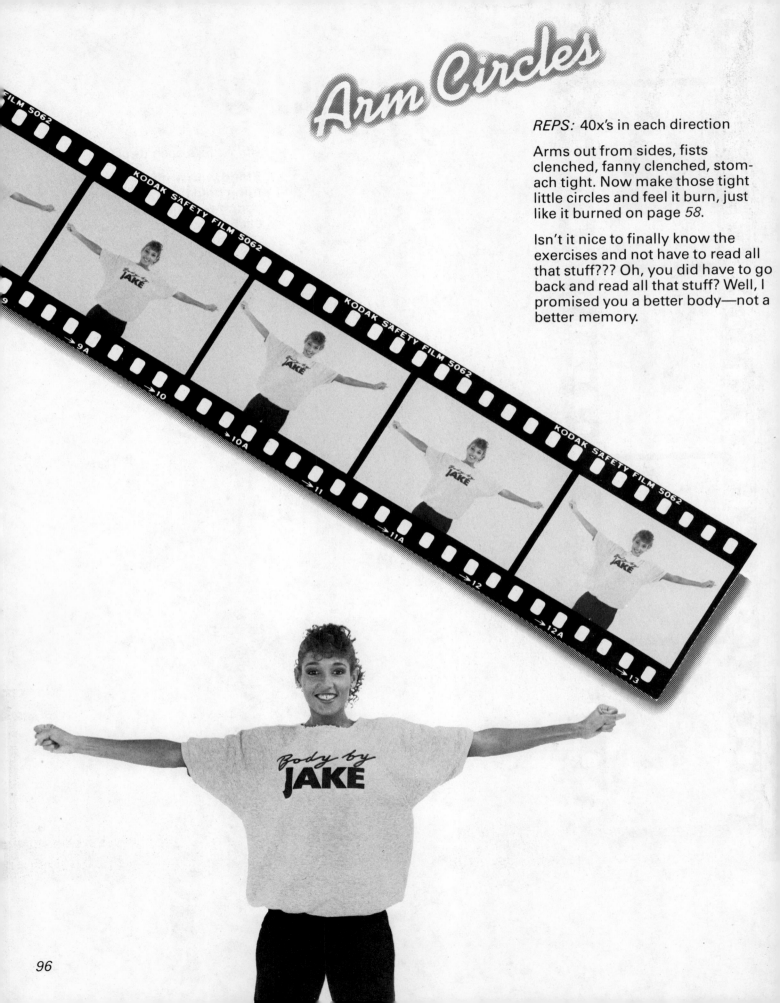

REPS: 40x's in each direction

Arms out from sides, fists clenched, fanny clenched, stomach tight. Now make those tight little circles and feel it burn, just like it burned on page *58*.

Isn't it nice to finally know the exercises and not have to read all that stuff??? Oh, you did have to go back and read all that stuff? Well, I promised you a better body—not a better memory.

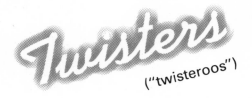

Twisters

("twisteroos")

REPS: 40x's—full twist is one count

Stand as shown and gimme the old twisteroos WITHOUT moving from the waist down unless you move back to page *59* to see the original Twisters.

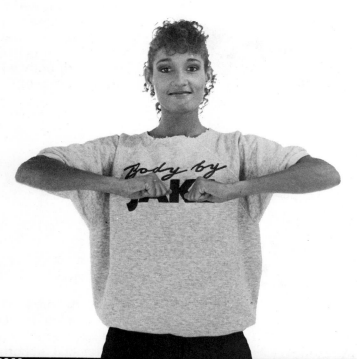

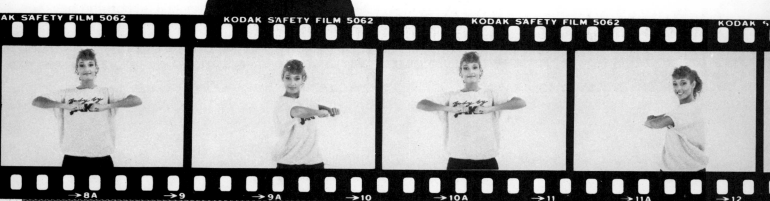

✳Variation from previous chapter.

Broomstick Twisters *

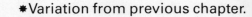

REPS: 40x's

VARIATION!!!! I wanna keep you on your toes!

Hold the broomstick IN FRONT OF YOUR CHEST instead of behind your neck, and then proceed. If you can't proceed then return to page *61* so you can proceed!

Stand as shown with the broomstick held tight in front and then twist as usual. Make sure your hips don't move and your focus is directly ahead with your head not moving.

Broomstick Side Stretches

REPS: 25x's

Back to the old position of the broomstick behind your back and over your upper arm like the last chapter. Is it all coming back to you? If not see page *61*.

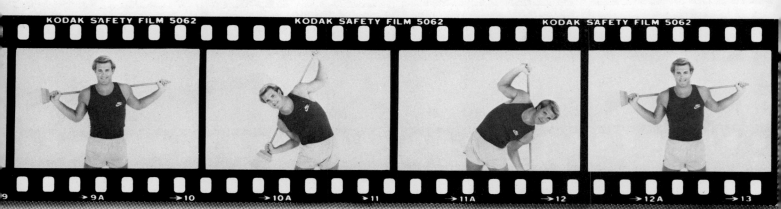

Broomstick Single Side Stretches

REPS: 25x's

Keep the broomstick where it is and give me the same thing only in one count on each side like you did on page *62.*

Bent Over Broomstick Twisters

REPS: 40x's

Keep the broomstick where it is and bend over! If you've forgotten this exercise, straighten back up and read page *62.*

With your back flat and keeping your head stationary...gimme 40 full Twisters in 15 seconds!

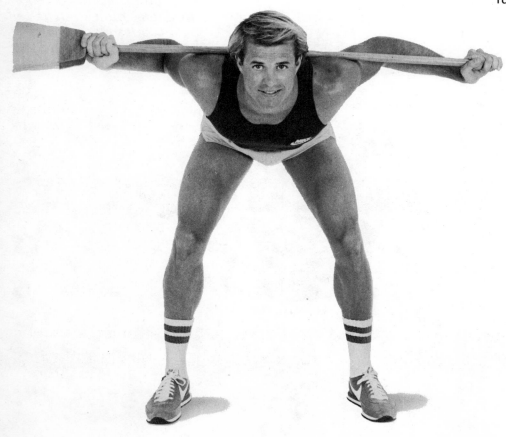

✱ Variation from previous chapter.

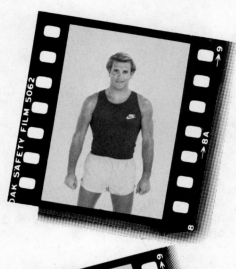

Side Stretches

REPS: 15x's each set

1. Arms at sides–EVERYTHING held tight!

2. Reach arm down one leg while pulling other arm up toward armpit alternating sides. Both sides together count as 1, 2, 3; 1, 2, 3; 2, 2, 3; 2, 2, 3; etc.

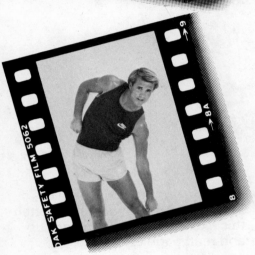

Single Side Stretches

REPS: 15x's each set

1. Keep body in same position and do single count stretches alternating sides while counting 1, and; 2, and; 3, and; etc.

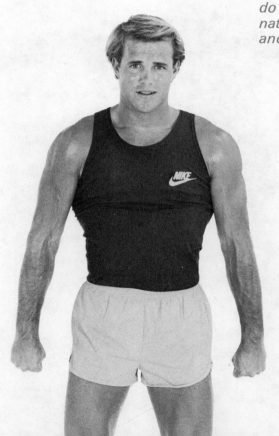

Over Head Side Stretches

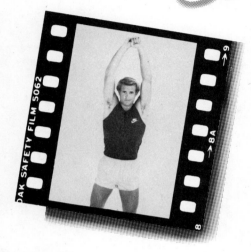

REPS: 15x's each set

1. *Arms stretched over head with thumbs hooked and body held tight.*

2. *Stretch side to side counting as above: 1, 2, 3; 1, 2, 3; 2, 2, 3; 2, 2, 3; etc.*

Single Over Head Side Stretches

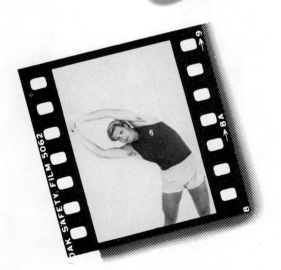

REPS: 15x's each set

1. *Keep body in same position and do single count over head stretches while counting 1, and; 2, and; 3, and....*

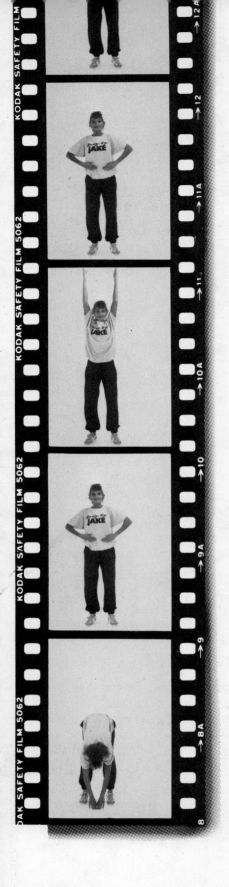

Toe Touches

REPS: 25x's

Just like before on page *65*—only more!!!

Runs #1

REPS: 25x's

Stay down, stay streamlined, stay in there!

VARIATION COMING UP—
VARIATION COMING UP—
VARIATION COMING UP

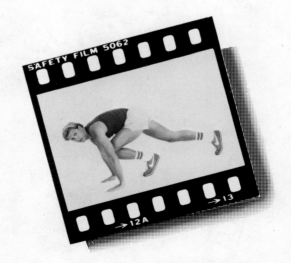

Advanced Butt Burners #1 ✳

REPS: 25x's each leg

1. Get down on hands and knees, EXTEND RIGHT LEG OUT TO THE SIDE, PERPENDICULAR TO YOUR BODY.

2. With foot flexed and leg held tight, raise and lower leg, WITHOUT LETTING IT TOUCH THE FLOOR.

   Gimme 25 on each leg and keep that leg extended to the side.

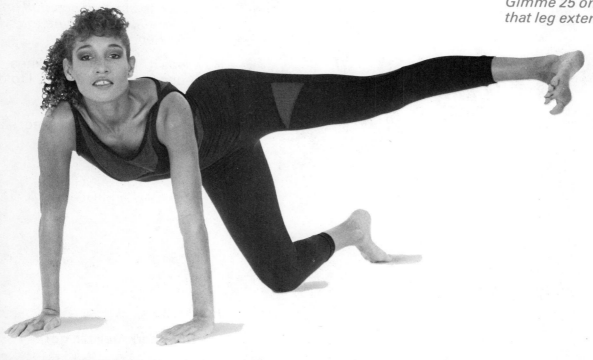

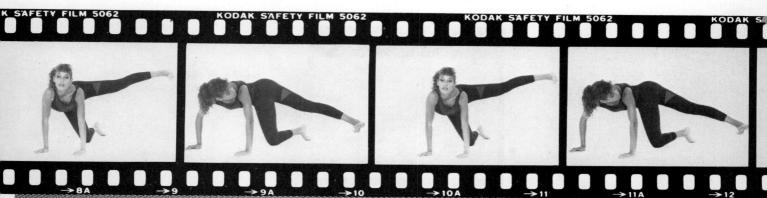

Big Boy Push-Ups #1

FOR: Toning and strengthening upper body
REPS: 5x's
TIME: 5 seconds

BIG TIME!!!!

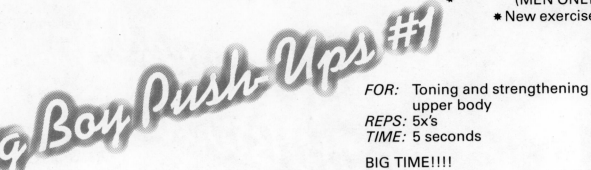

1. Lie face down on the floor with your hands flat beside your shoulders and legs extended full out with your weight on your toes.

2. Push with your hands until your arms are straight—but don't lock-out.

3. Return to starting position until you're almost touching the floor. Repeat.

How was it? Did doing the knee Push-ups for a month help? I told you so!!!

Runs #2

REPS: 25x's

On your mark, get set, go!

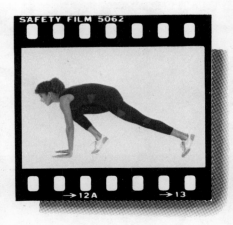

Advanced Inner Thigh

REPS: 25x's each side

1. Lie on the floor the same as the old Inner Thigh exercise on page 70.

2. The difference is that I want you to HOLD THE BOTTOM LEG AS FAR TOWARD THE REAR AS YOU CAN. And keep it there for all 25!

Don't tell me you can't feel a difference.

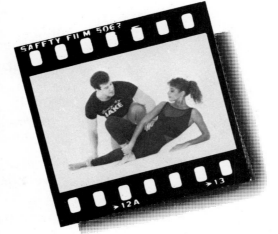

(MEN ONLY)

Big Boy Push-Ups #2

All ready big fella??!!

REPS: 5x's

Make sure you keep your back straight and touch your chest, not your chin, to the floor.

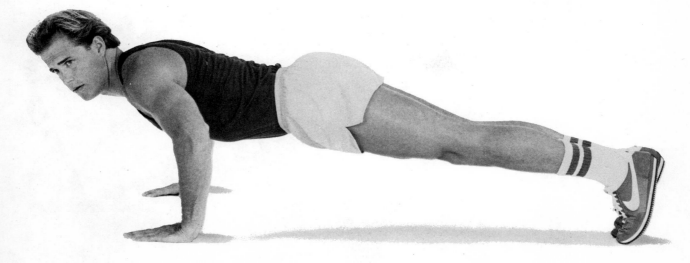

Combination Sitters

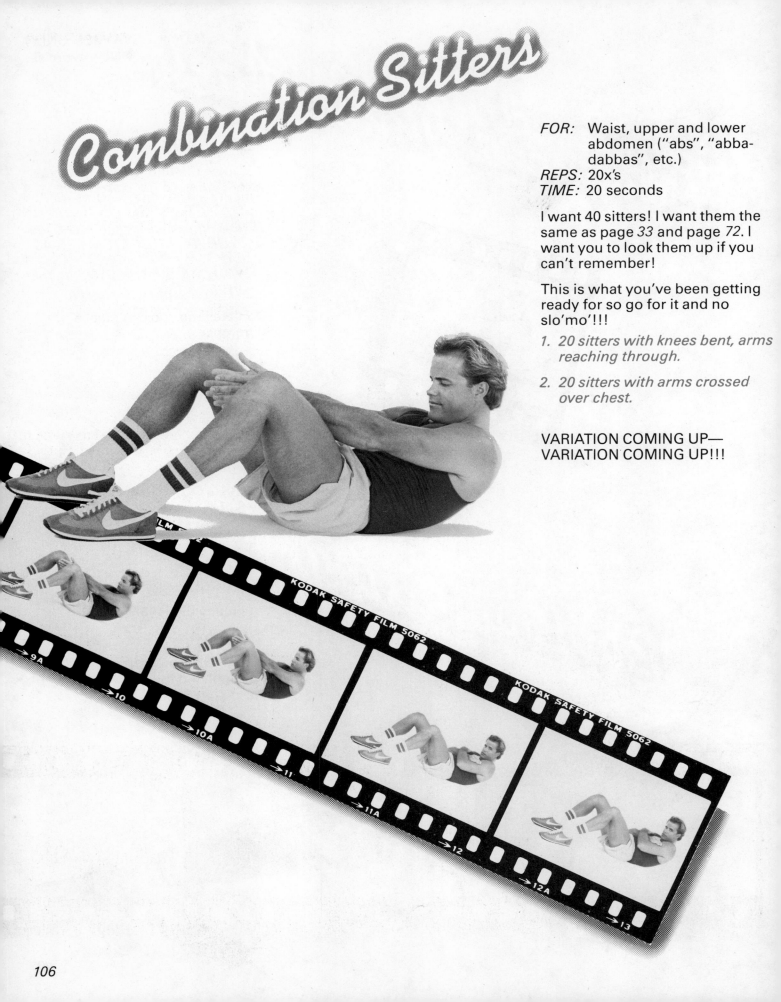

FOR: Waist, upper and lower abdomen ("abs", "abba-dabbas", etc.)
REPS: 20x's
TIME: 20 seconds

I want 40 sitters! I want them the same as page *33* and page *72*. I want you to look them up if you can't remember!

This is what you've been getting ready for so go for it and no slo'mo'!!!

1. *20 sitters with knees bent, arms reaching through.*

2. *20 sitters with arms crossed over chest.*

VARIATION COMING UP—
VARIATION COMING UP!!!

Advanced Leg Raises *

REPS: 20x's for each set

SETS: 3

These are the same leg movements as the other leg lifts, (on page *73*) but you should be UP ON YOUR HANDS for all three sets.

1. *Sit propped up on your hands with elbows slightly bent.*

2. *First set, pull your legs in toward your chest then out.*

3. *Second set, still resting on hands, do the Scissors as shown on page 74.*

4. *Third set, Baby Runs while still on hands as shown on page 75.*

Those are tough!!! But stick with it. Your stomach won't only tighten up but your balance will be terrific!

Let's do another set of Runs before we get to the WEIGHTS!!!

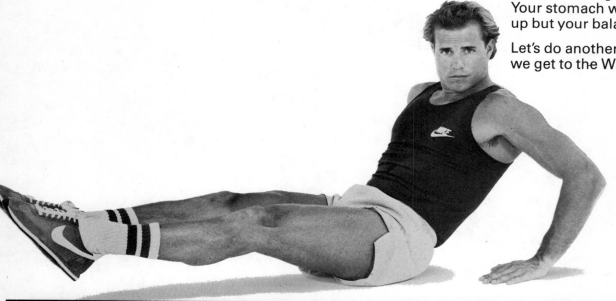

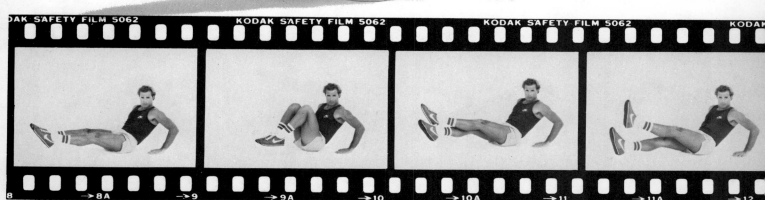

Runs #3

REPS: 25x's

Going, going, gone!

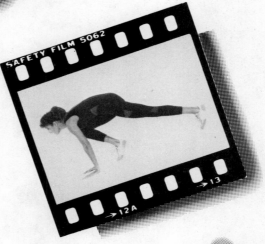

(WOMEN ONLY)

Advanced Butt Burners #2

REPS: 25x's each leg

You should be past burning at this point and into smokin' em!

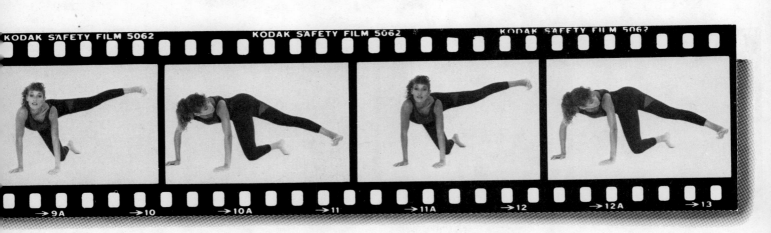

Big Boy Push-Ups #3

REPS: 5x's

If at first you don't succeed . . .

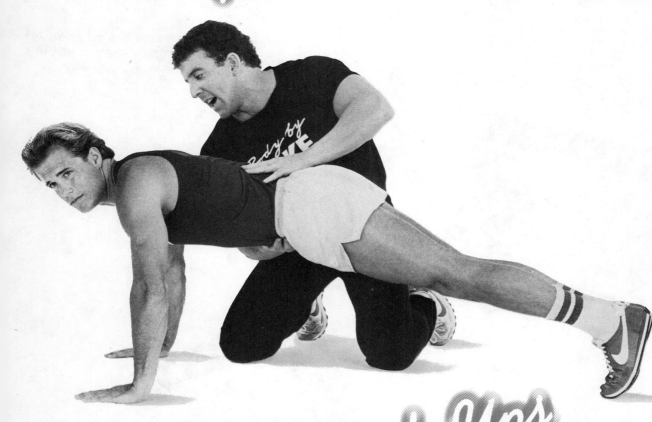

Push-Ups

(EVERYBODY)

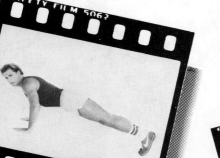

REPS: Ladies: 15x's
Men: 25x's
(it'll be a cinch!)

Up, down. Up, down. Up, down . . .

Not only are we getting closer to the weights . . . we're getting closer to the end!

Let's stretch out and get ready!

Door Jamb Stretch

REPS: 15 counts on each side
SETS: 2

Single arm stretch like on page *79* and don't skimp on the time trying to hurry to the weights!

HERE WE GO!!!

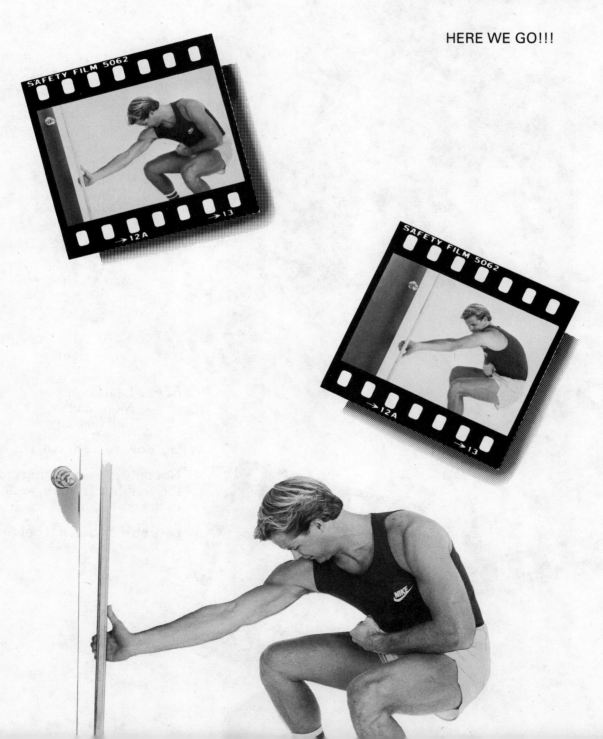

Two Arm Dumbbell Press Or 50 Arm Circles

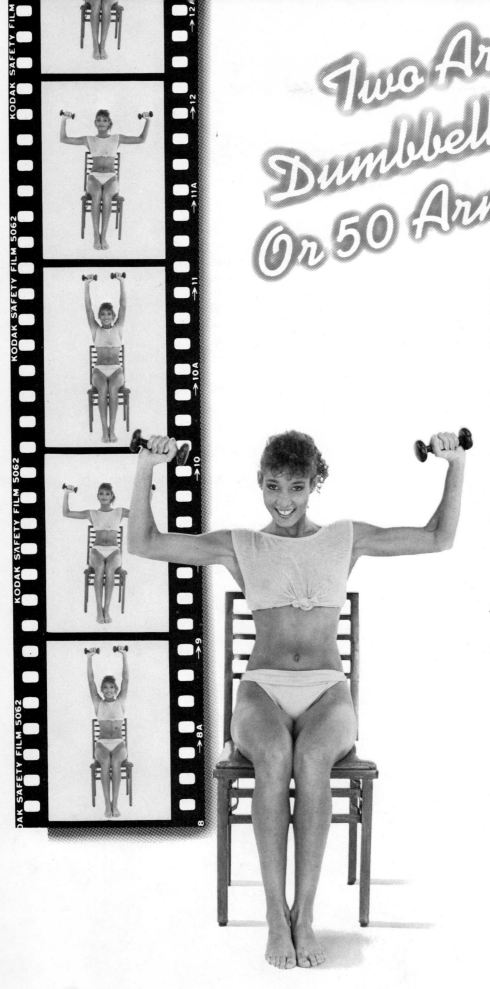

First we're gonna do Two Arm Dumbbell Presses. If you aren't working with weights yet I want you to SUBSTITUTE 50 ARM CIRCLES IN EACH DIRECTION FROM page *58*.

FOR: Firming and shaping the front and sides of shoulders and back of upper arms

REPS: 10x's

WEIGHT: Women: 2-3 lbs.
             Men: 10 lbs.

TIME: 10 seconds

1. *Sit in chair with your back touching back of the chair, feet flat on floor, a dumbbell in each hand, arm raised shoulder height and elbows flexed.*

2. *Press both dumbbells overhead while inhaling.*

3. *Lower dumbbells back to starting position while exhaling.*

I know they seem easy now but by the tenth press wait and see!

Bicep Curl Or Door Knob Bicep Curls *

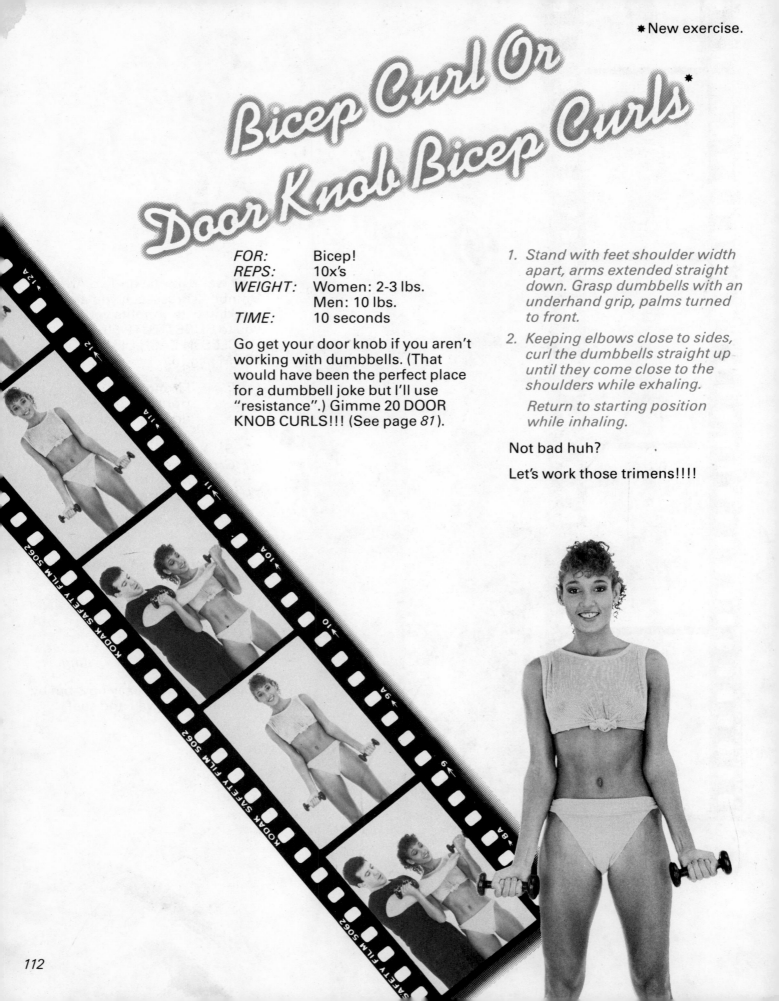

FOR: Bicep!
REPS: 10x's
WEIGHT: Women: 2-3 lbs.
　　　　　 Men: 10 lbs.
TIME: 10 seconds

Go get your door knob if you aren't working with dumbbells. (That would have been the perfect place for a dumbbell joke but I'll use "resistance".) Gimme 20 DOOR KNOB CURLS!!! (See page *81*).

1. Stand with feet shoulder width apart, arms extended straight down. Grasp dumbbells with an underhand grip, palms turned to front.

2. Keeping elbows close to sides, curl the dumbbells straight up until they come close to the shoulders while exhaling.

   Return to starting position while inhaling.

Not bad huh?

Let's work those trimens!!!!

112

Tricep Push-Up

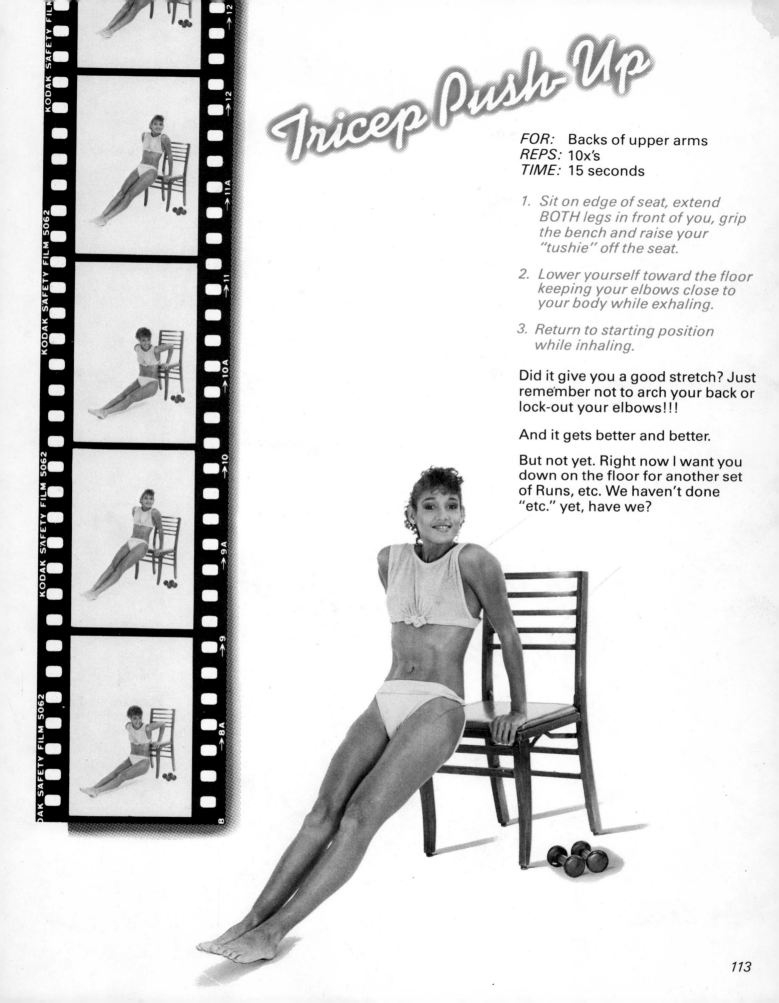

FOR: Backs of upper arms
REPS: 10x's
TIME: 15 seconds

1. Sit on edge of seat, extend BOTH legs in front of you, grip the bench and raise your "tushie" off the seat.

2. Lower yourself toward the floor keeping your elbows close to your body while exhaling.

3. Return to starting position while inhaling.

Did it give you a good stretch? Just remember not to arch your back or lock-out your elbows!!!

And it gets better and better.

But not yet. Right now I want you down on the floor for another set of Runs, etc. We haven't done "etc." yet, have we?

Runs #4

REPS: 25x's

These seem pretty easy after that, don't they. I mean they're almost relaxing!

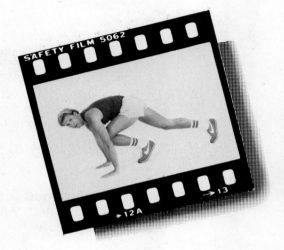

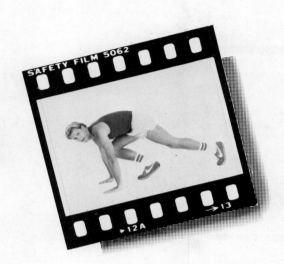

Advanced Inner Thigh #2

REPS: 25x's each leg

Remember to keep forcing the leg you're working back with the foot flexed as shown.
Remember to look up "how to" on page *105* if you can't remember how to.

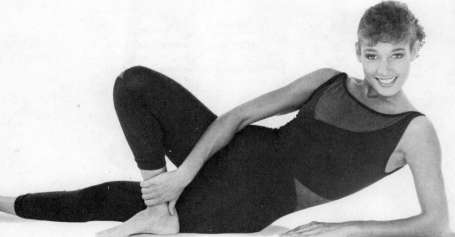

114

Big Boy Push-Ups #4

REPS: 5x's

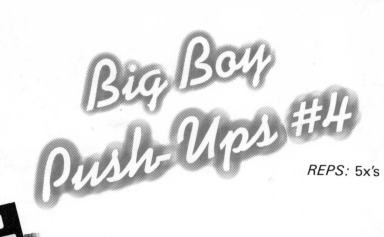

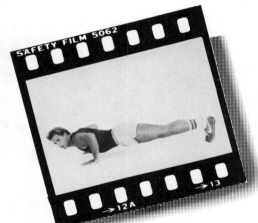

* Variation from previous chapter.

Broomstick Lunges *

Do lunges as before but this time hold a broomstick behind your shoulders.

Remember not to let that back leg near the floor and keep your speed up!

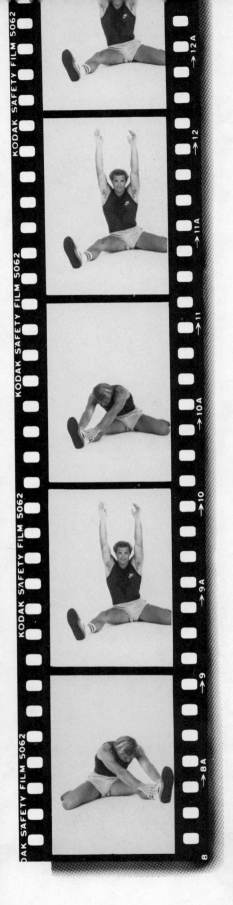

Hurdles
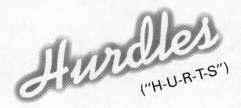
("H-U-R-T-S")

REPS: 15 counts each leg

Don't force the reach. Don't force the stretch. Don't forget to look this up on page *88* if you've forgotten. Breath deeply and recover!

Wishbone Stretch
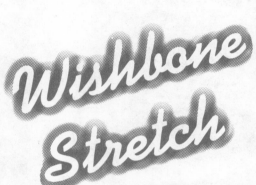

REPS: 15 counts

Open those legs and let loose! This is it. Again, don't force the reach, don't force the stretch. But lemme ask you: can't you stretch farther than you did a month ago? I knew it!

Bonus! Stay where you are for a second. The coach here wants to talk to you before you shower up!

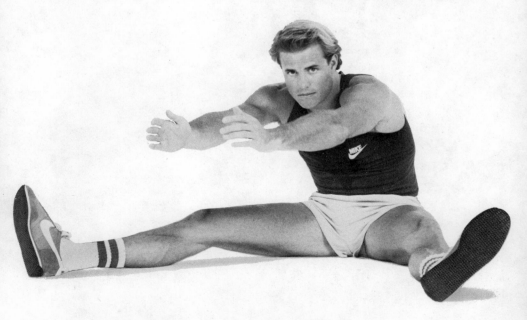

I want to tell you a little more about "locking-out". Now that you've had a run through with the instructions for this chapter, you probably understand what I was trying to tell you. When you "lock-out," or push your joints, like elbows and knees, in the opposite direction, you're really putting a lot of stress on tendons and ligaments that hold your bones together. Even though "locking-out" may make you feel stronger, you're not. Learn to straighten your arms and legs without locking your elbows and knees whether working with weights or just exercising.

On the other hand, don't overstretch a joint either. Your knees and elbows don't have any muscles of their own. It's the muscles around them that give them their strength. Don't bend your knees or elbows beyond the point where these muscles can control and support the movement. So, watch yourself when you bend your knees on Lunges or straighten your arms on Push-ups.

I guess that's enough of a lecture huh? Just stick in there, you're doing great!

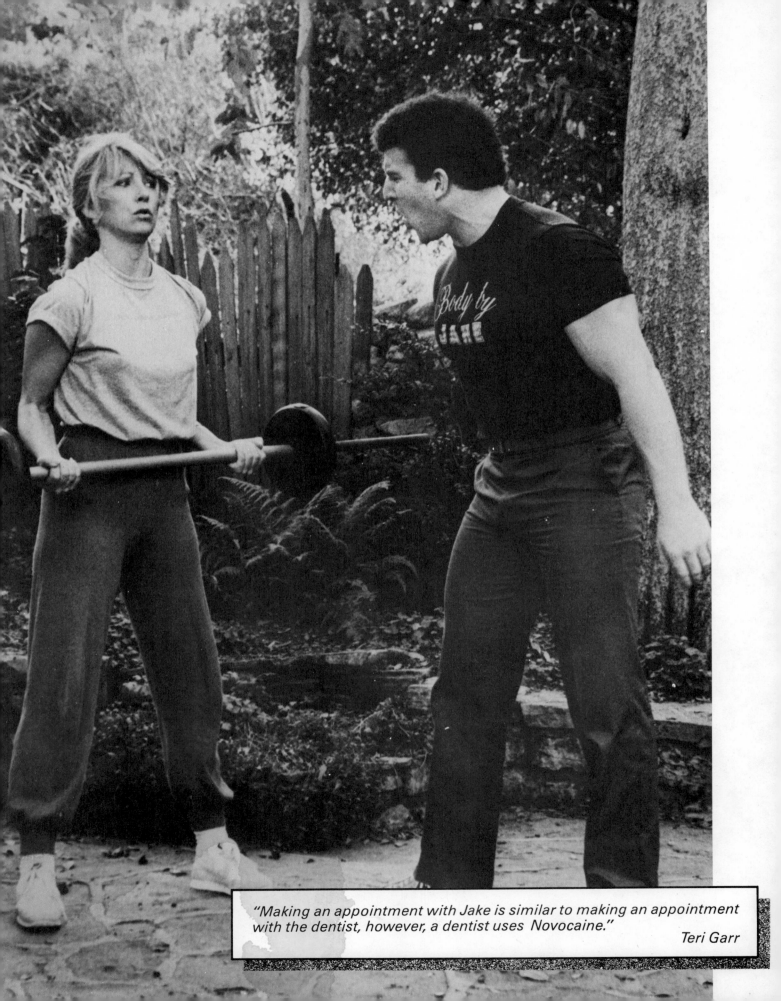

"Making an appointment with Jake is similar to making an appointment with the dentist, however, a dentist uses Novocaine."

Teri Garr

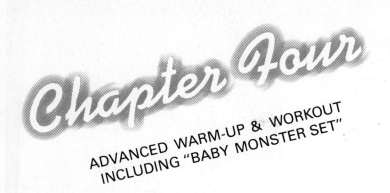

Chapter Four

ADVANCED WARM-UP & WORKOUT INCLUDING "BABY MONSTER SET"

Well, by now we've built up your strength and stamina and you should be well on your way to a well-toned body. But, there's one thing I haven't mentioned. FAT! Are you still FAT!? Y'now, behind every big behind there's a little behind just dying to get out. If you don't believe me... go look in the mirror. How BIG is it??? Just what I thought. But don't take it personally. It's just that most people don't realize that for every ten years after we're grown up we get 10% less activity and need 10% less food. So, if you've been eating like a teenager and exercising like someone your age should... it's just not good enough. Generally, if you want to lose a pound you gotta eat 3500 fewer calories. This means that it will probably take longer than a day to lose that weight.

Combining exercise with diet means that you'll be burning fat while gaining lean muscle tissue. But this is only true if the exercise keeps your heart pumpin' the way the Steinfeld Sprints do. So, in this chapter you get to do the Baby Monster Set. It's called Baby Monster Set for two reasons. One is that you'll sweat like a monster and the other is that it's TOUGH. In this set you do runs in between every exercise! But if you want to burn fat you gotta do it. You can help it along with what you eat too.

I've always been interested in building muscle and the kind of diet that does this is one that's high in protein and low in carbohydrates. This kind of diet is not for everyone and before you start any kind of diet you should check with your doctor. I'm also not saying that "carbs" are bad. It's just that when you exercise, your body burns those quick energy "carbs" stored in muscles first and it's only after the first ten or fifteen minutes of burning these that your body starts to burn the long term energy stores of fat. So, choose your carbohydrates carefully. You want to eat the kind that are complex and harder to burn rather than the kind in ice cream sundaes. And when you're considering that ice cream sundae, consider this while your at it: to burn it off will require 3½ hours of running, 4½ hours of swimming or 10 hours of climbing stairs!!!

Besides the extra Runs in this chapter, which couldn't hurt even if you aren't trying to lose weight, most of you are probably working with weights. As you progress, there are additional reps and sets with weights but not any added weight. You can also increase the reps in the exercises, just make sure your workout doesn't exceed thirty minutes. It doesn't need to.

So like I keep telling you... let's get lean and mean!

ADVANCED WARM-UP & WORKOUT INTRODUCING "THE BABY MONSTER SET"

- READ CAREFULLY BEFORE ATTEMPTING PROGRAM
- WOMEN • 2-3 LBS.   • IF TOO DIFFICULT RETURN TO CHAPTER THREE
- MEN • 10 LBS   • ADD REPETITIONS AT OWN DISCRETION

CHAPTER FOUR

EXERCISES	Workout 1 REPS	Workout 1 U DID	Workout 2 REPS	Workout 2 U DID	Workout 3 REPS	Workout 3 U DID	Workout 4 REPS	Workout 4 U DID	Workout 5 REPS	Workout 5 U DID	GOAL
BIG STRETCH	10										
HEAD ROLLS	5										
* ARM CIRCLES/ WEIGHTS	50/25										
TWISTERS/WEIGHTS	50/25										
BROOMSTICK: TWISTERS	50										
SIDE STRETCHES	30										
SINGLE SIDE STRETCHES	30										
BENT OVER TWISTERS	50										
*SIDE: WEIGHTS STRETCHES	20										
SINGLES	20										
OVER HEAD	20										
SINGLE OVER HEAD	20										
TOE TOUCHES	35										
RUNS #1	50										
LUNGES/RUNS #2 (w/Broomstick)	20/25										
ADVANCED INNER THIGH/RUNS #3	25/25										
*BODY BURNERS/ RUNS #4	25/25										
ADVANCED BUTT BURNERS/RUNS #5	25/25										
WISHBONE STRETCH	25		(HOLD FOR 25 COUNTS IN EACH POSITION)								
HURDLES	25		(HOLD FOR 25 COUNTS EACH SIDE)								
STANDING DUMBBELL PRESS/RUNS # 6	10/25										
*BICEP CURL/RUNS # 7	10/25										
*DUMBBELL SIDE LATERALS/RUNS #8	10/25										
*TRICEP EXTENSION/RUNS #9	10/50										

(Women Only)

	Workout 1 REPS	Workout 1 U DID	Workout 2 REPS	Workout 2 U DID	Workout 3 REPS	Workout 3 U DID	Workout 4 REPS	Workout 4 U DID	Workout 5 REPS	Workout 5 U DID	GOAL
BICEP CURL	10										
RUNS #2	50										
*TWO CHAIR PUSH-UPS #1	5										
RUNS #3	50										
STANDING DUMBBELL PRESSES	10										
RUNS #4	50										
DUMBBELL SIDE LATERALS	10										
RUNS #5	50										
*SHOULDER DUMBBELL PRESSES	10										
RUNS #6	50										
TWO CHAIR PUSH-UPS	5										
RUNS #7	50										
*TRICEP EXTENSION	10										
RUNS #8	50										
*LUNGES	10										
RUNS #9	50										
*SQUATS	25										
RUNS #10	50										
BIG BOY PUSH-UPS	5/25										
*LEG RAISES: IN/OUTS	50										
SCISSORS	50										
BABY RUNS	50										
RUNS #11	50										
*BIG CRUNCH	50										
WISHBONE STRETCH	25		COUNTS								
HURDLES	25		COUNTS								
EGG ROLL	1										

(Everybody)

Everybody works together warming-up and then we'll split up for the Baby Monster Set

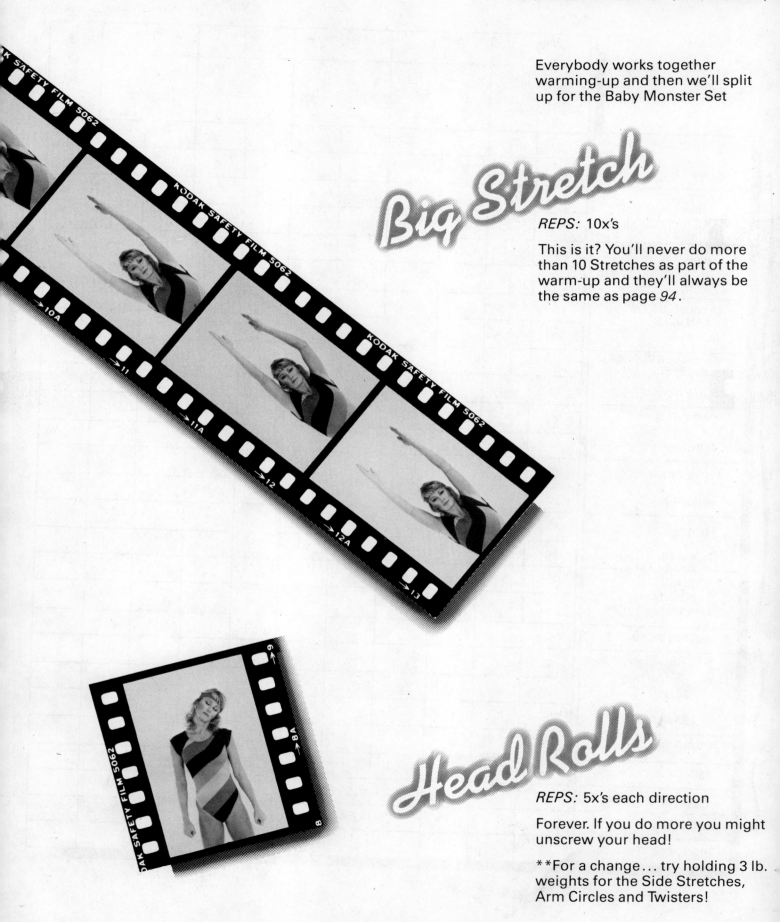

Big Stretch

REPS: 10x's

This is it? You'll never do more than 10 Stretches as part of the warm-up and they'll always be the same as page *94*.

Head Rolls

REPS: 5x's each direction

Forever. If you do more you might unscrew your head!

**For a change... try holding 3 lb. weights for the Side Stretches, Arm Circles and Twisters!

Stretches:

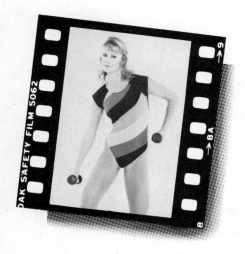

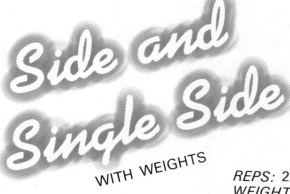

Side and Single Side

WITH WEIGHTS

REPS: 20x's
WEIGHT: 3 lbs.

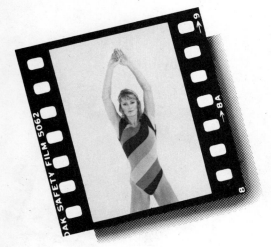

Over Head

REPS: 20x's

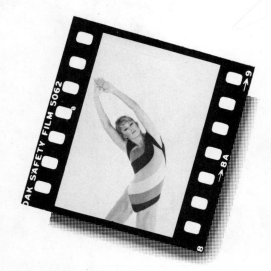

Single Over Head

REPS: 20x's

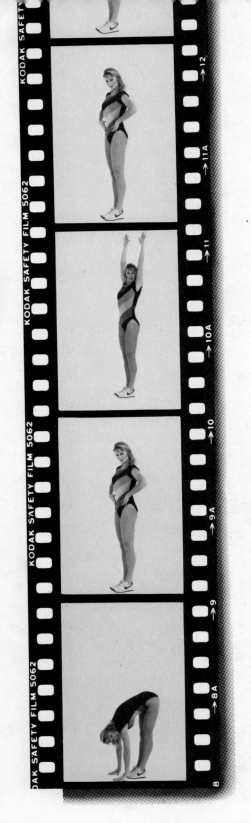

Toe Touches

REPS: 35x's

Hips and up, Hips and down, Hips and up, Hips and down, Hip, Hip, Hooray!

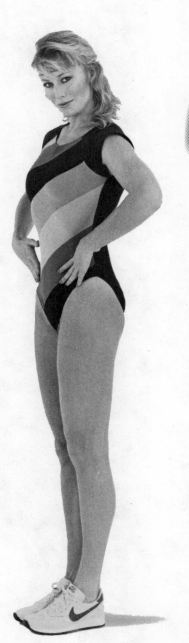

Runs #1

REPS: 50x's

Giddy-up!

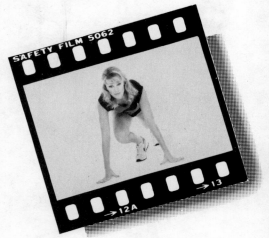

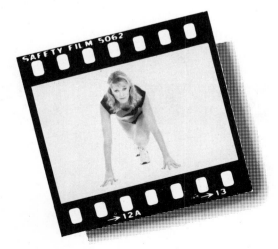

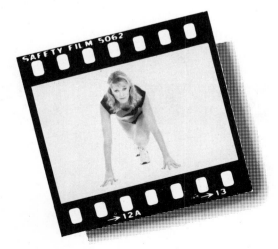

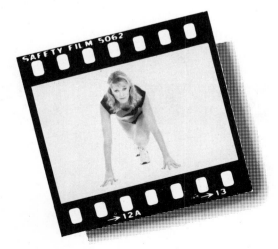

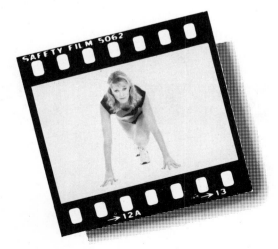

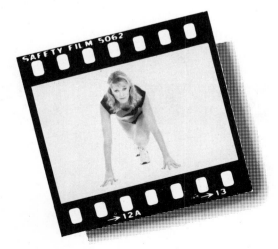

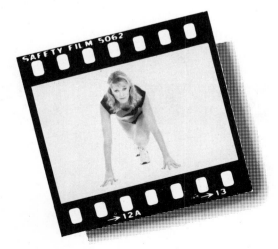

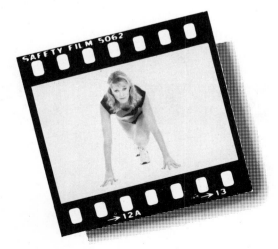

Okay ladies, get ready to smoke 'em!!!

Don't stop in between these exercises. If it is really and I mean really, too much for you, then drop all the numbers back by ten but keep the runs in between.

There's something else very important—read through this program before you attempt it. If you have to stop and look up *any* exercises you haven't learned the exercises well enough to do the Baby Monster Set. This set requires constant movement, you know what I mean? No slo' mo'! Speed and maximum exertion! Okay, now *read* on.

And then turn to page *145* to rejoin the men for the rest of the workout.

Gentlemen proceed to page *136* for your own Baby Monster Set.

Lunges With Broomstick Behind Shoulders

REPS: 20x's each side

Runs #2

REPS: 25x's

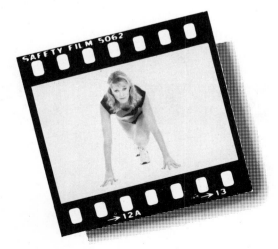

Advanced Inner Thigh

REPS: 25x's each side

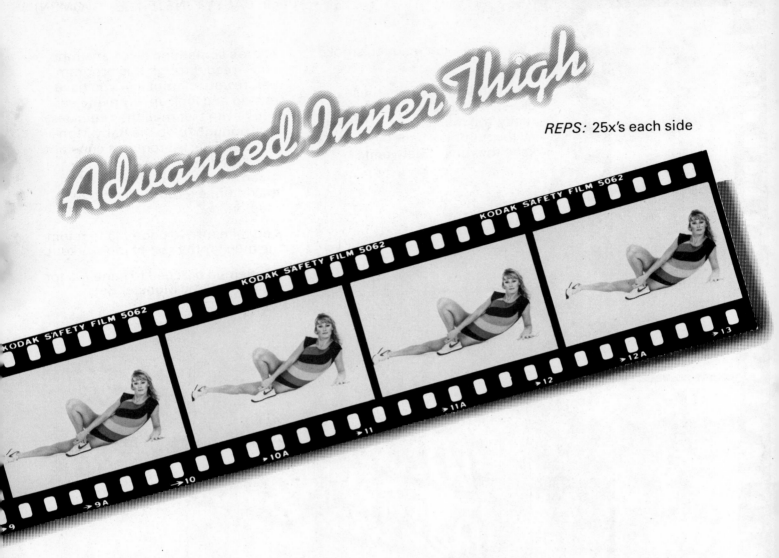

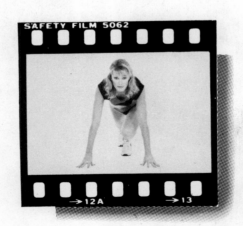

Runs #3

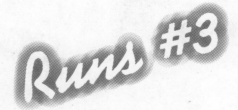

REPS: 25x's

Body Burners

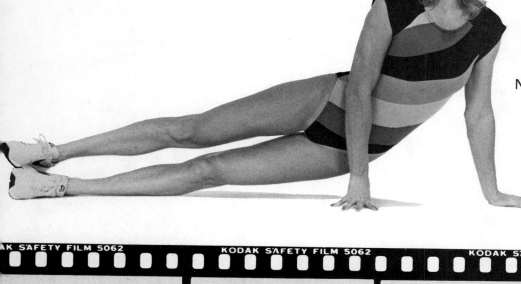

FOR: Strengthening upper body and "tushie".
REPS: 25x's each side
TIME: 25 seconds

1. Lie on your side, supporting your weight on hands placed in front with elbows straight.

   Raise and lower upper leg. Change sides and repeat with opposite leg.

   Gimme 25 smokers on each side.

   Now stay down there and run!

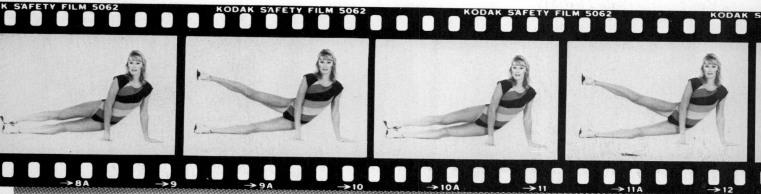

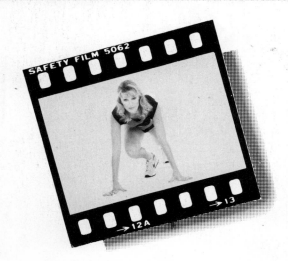

Runs #4

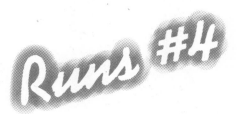

REPS: 25x's

Advanced Butt Burners

REPS: 25x's each leg

Keep that leg up and out to the side with that foot flexed!!!

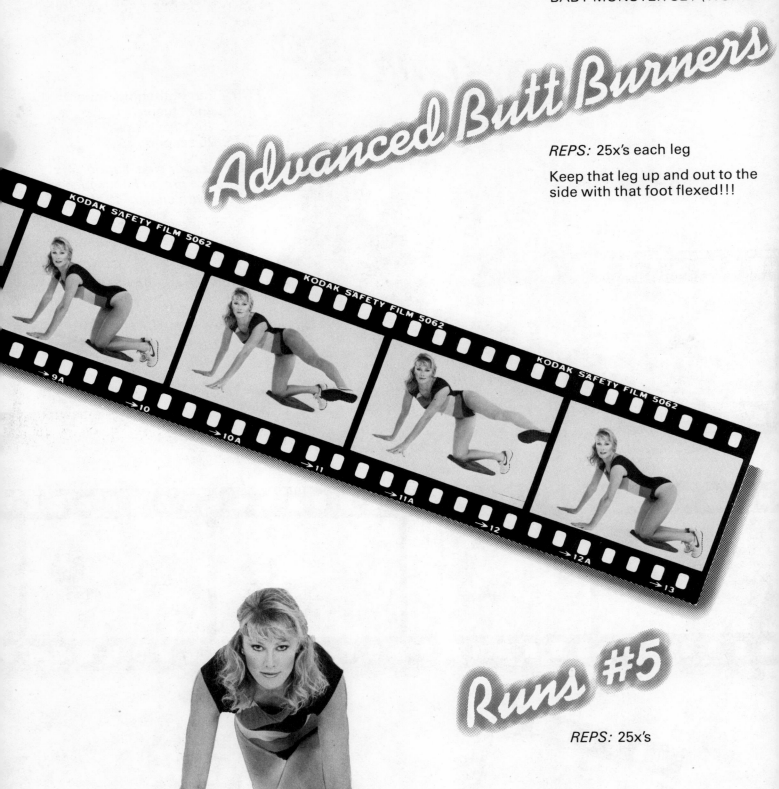

Runs #5

REPS: 25x's

Wishbone Stretch

REPS: Hold for 25 counts in each position—left, right, center

You deserve it.

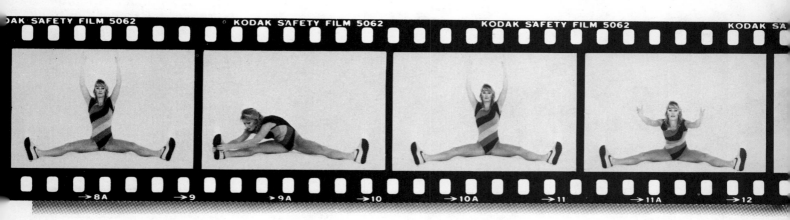

Hurdles

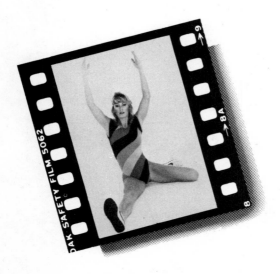

REPS: Hold for 25 counts each side

Are you sweating like a monster?

We've cooked the lower body... let's move on up!

Get those weights!

Standing Dumbbell Press

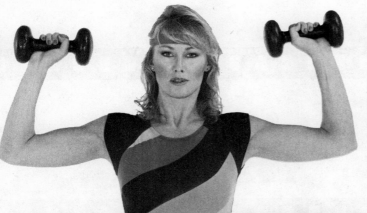

FOR: Strengthening shoulders
REPS: 10x's
WEIGHT: 2-3 lbs.
TIME: 15 seconds

1. *Stand straight, feet shoulder width apart. Grasp a dumbbell in each hand, shoulder height with elbows bent and palms facing front.*

2. *Press both dumbbells over head while exhaling.*

3. *Lower dumbbells back to starting position while inhaling.*

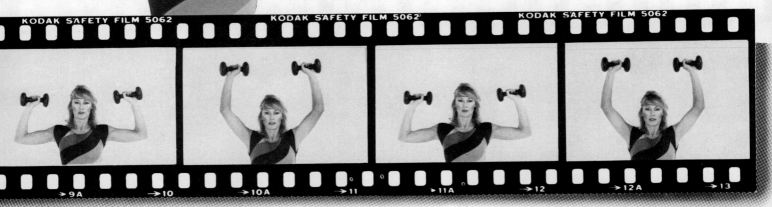

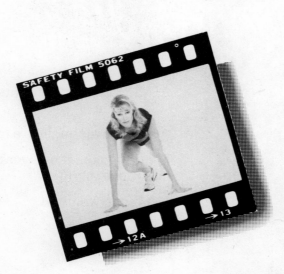

Runs # 6

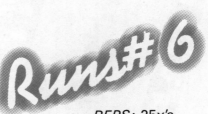

REPS: 25x's

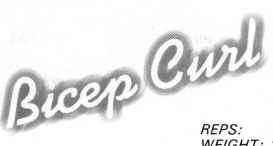

Bicep Curl

REPS: 10x's
WEIGHT: 2-3 lbs.

1. *Stand with feet shoulder width apart, grasp weights with an underhand grip keeping elbows close to waist.*

2. *Still keeping elbows close to your body, lift weight toward shoulders.*

3. *Return slowly to starting position.*

Don't lock-out on the full extension and don't arch your back!

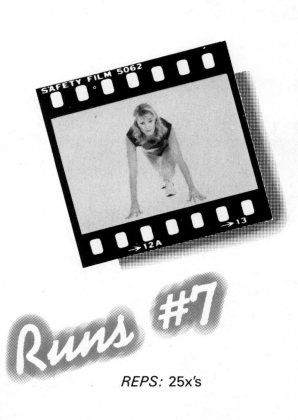

Runs #7

REPS: 25x's

Dumbbell Side Laterals*

REPS: 10x's
WEIGHT: 2-3 lbs.

This is new! Read these instructions carefully. The life you save may be your own!

1. *Stand erect with feet about 12 inches apart holding a dumbbell in each hand arms hanging down with palms facing thighs.*

2. *Keeping arms straight, raise the dumbbells upward with slightly bent arms to shoulder height.*

   Return slowly to starting position.

Do this exercise and you'll never have saggy underarms or flabby armpits!

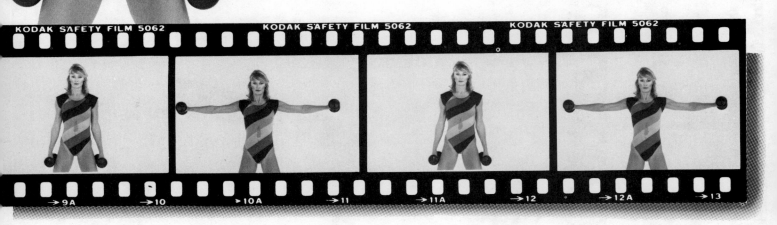

KODAK SAFETY FILM 5062

→9A →10 →10A →11 →11A →12 →12A →13

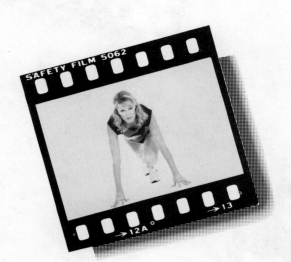

SAFETY FILM 5062

→12A →13

Runs # 8

REPS: 25x's

Tricep Extension

REPS: 10x's
WEIGHT: 2-3 lbs.

1. Sitting in chair with feet flat on floor and back straight, hold one end of a dumbbell over head with both hands and arms extended.

2. Bend your elbows to bring the dumbbell down behind your head. Keep your elbows very close to your ears.

   Return to starting position.

Lean over, put those weights on the floor and STAY DOWN THERE and give me 50 runs.

Runs #9

REPS: 50x's

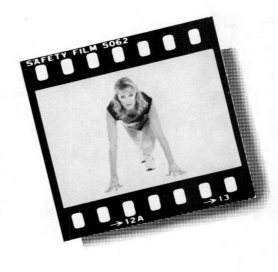

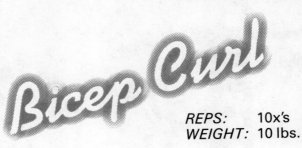

Bicep Curl

REPS: 10x's
WEIGHT: 10 lbs.

1. *Stand with feet shoulder width apart, arms hanging straight with a dumbbell in each hand—palms forward.*

2. *Keeping elbows close to body, raise dumbbells up to shoulders.*

3. *Return to a position of full extension.*

Don't lock-out on the full extension and don't arch your back!

(MEN)

Runs #2

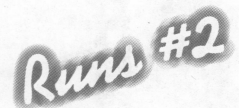

REPS: 50x's

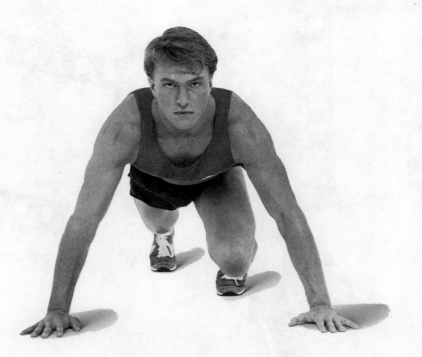

136

Two Chair Push-Ups #1

FOR: Strengthening upper body
REPS: 5x's
TIME: 10 seconds

This is real, I mean, REAL tough.

Position two chairs against wall so that the sides of the chairs are against the wall making sure they won't slip.

1. *Take the standard Push-up position with toes touching floor and each hand on a chair seat slightly wider than shoulders.*

2. *Lower until chest is slightly lower than chair seats and return to starting position.*

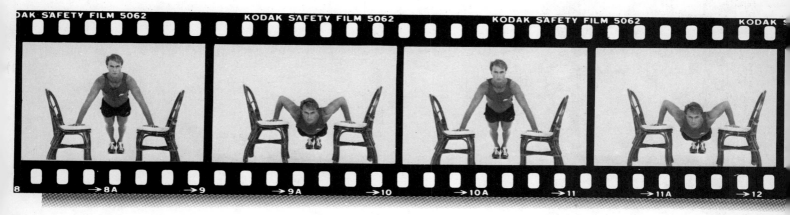

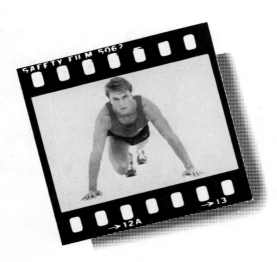

Runs #3

REPS: 50x's

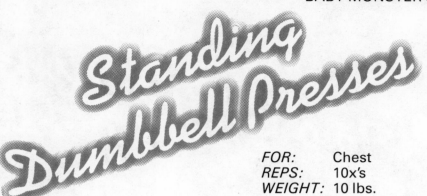

Standing Dumbbell Presses

FOR: Chest
REPS: 10x's
WEIGHT: 10 lbs.

1. Stand straight, feet shoulder width apart and arms raised to side with elbows bent—palms facing front.

2. Press both dumbbells over head while inhaling.

   Lower dumbbell back to starting position while exhaling.

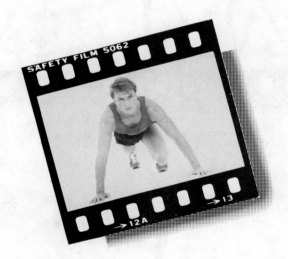

Runs #4

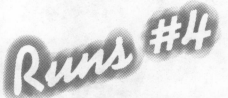

REPS: 50x's

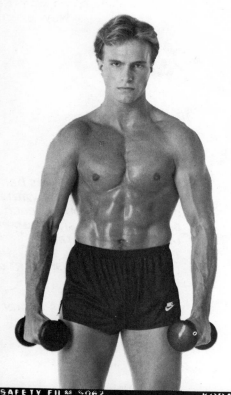

Dumbbell Side Laterals

REPS: 10x's
WEIGHT: 10 lbs.

1. *Stand erect with feet about 12 inches apart arms hanging straight down with a dumbbell in each hand, palms facing thighs.*

2. *Raise both arms, keeping the elbow slightly bent, to shoulder height.*

   Return slowly to starting position.

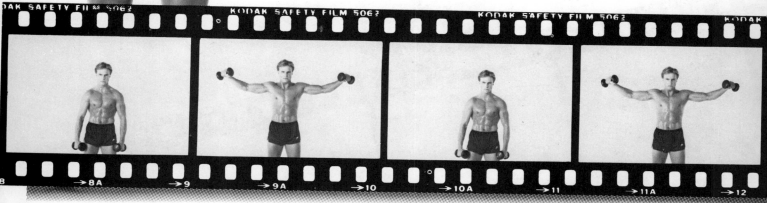

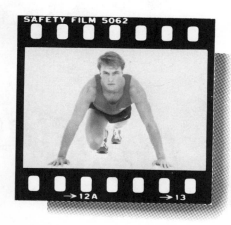

Runs #5

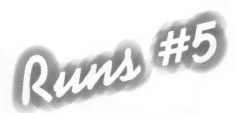

REPS: 50x's

Shoulder Dumbbell Presses*

FOR: Shoulders
REPS: 10x's
WEIGHT: 10 lbs.

1. Lie on back with knees bent and feet flat on floor, with a dumbbell grasped in each hand, extend arms to side with elbows bent and palms facing.

2. Press dumbbells straight up slowly.

Slowly return arms to starting position.

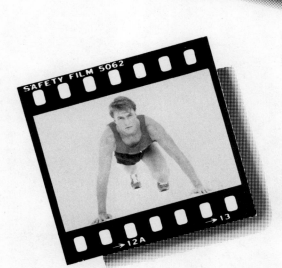

Runs # 6

REPS: 50x's

Two Chair Push-Ups #2

REPS: 5x's

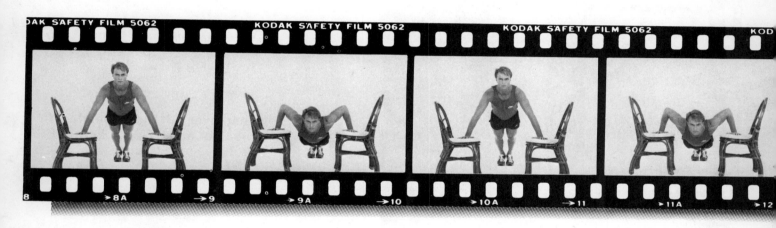

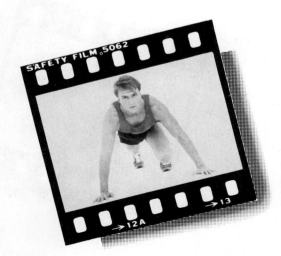

Runs #7

REPS: 50x's

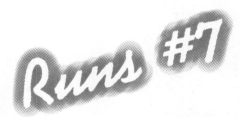

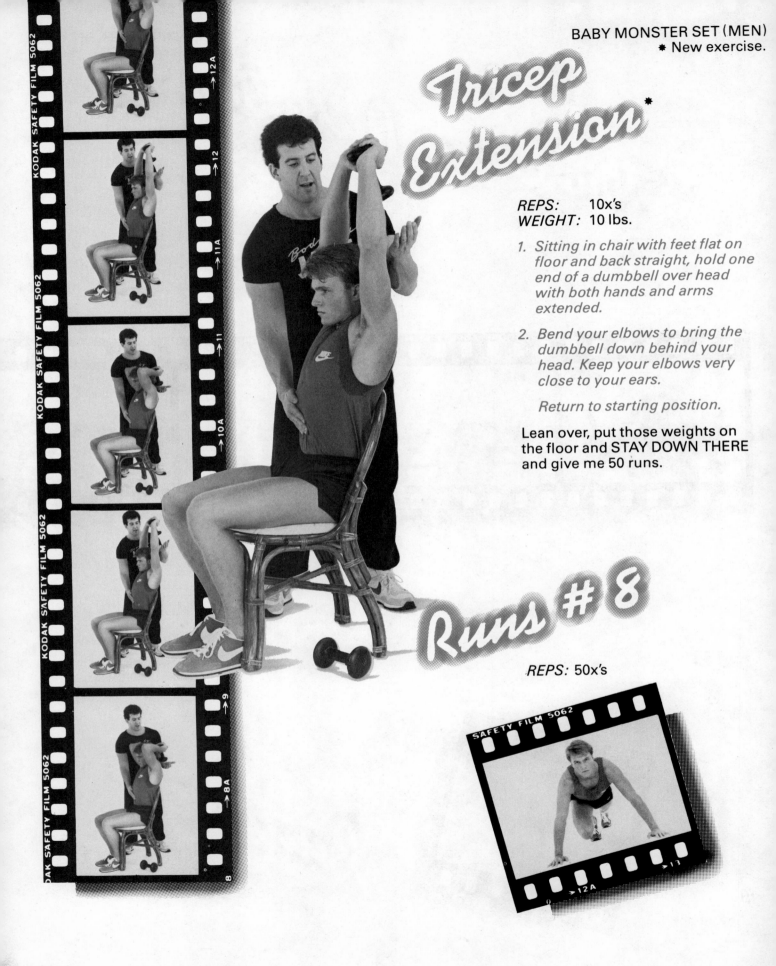

Tricep Extension *

REPS: 10x's
WEIGHT: 10 lbs.

1. Sitting in chair with feet flat on floor and back straight, hold one end of a dumbbell over head with both hands and arms extended.

2. Bend your elbows to bring the dumbbell down behind your head. Keep your elbows very close to your ears.

   Return to starting position.

Lean over, put those weights on the floor and STAY DOWN THERE and give me 50 runs.

Runs #8

REPS: 50x's

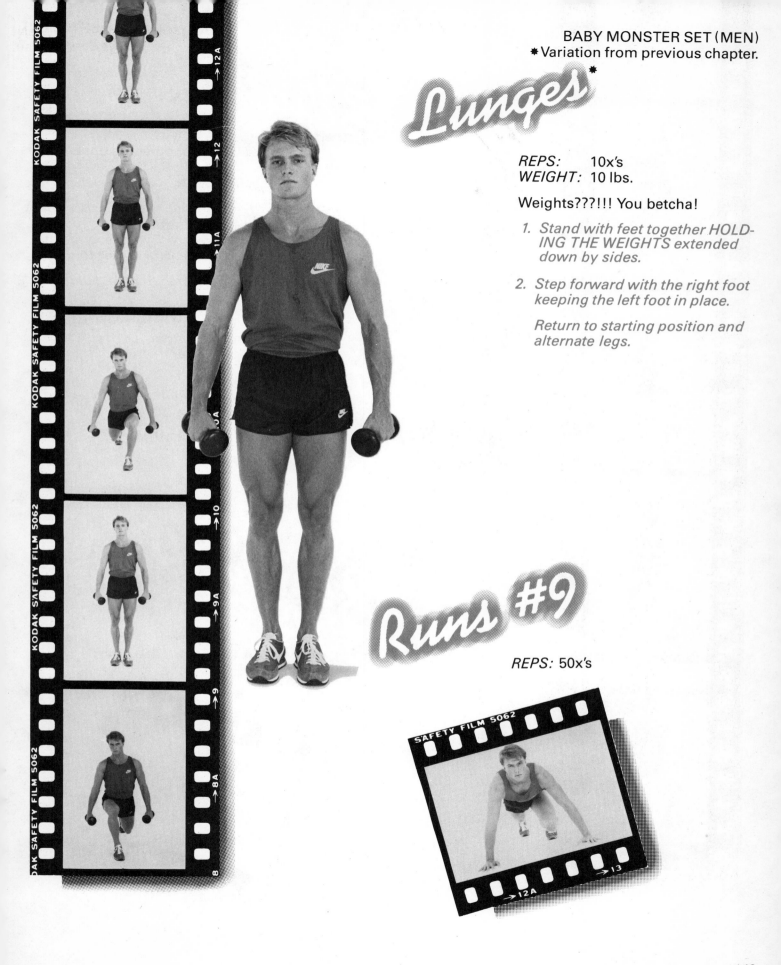

Lunges
*

REPS: 10x's
WEIGHT: 10 lbs.

Weights???!!! You betcha!

1. Stand with feet together HOLD-ING THE WEIGHTS extended down by sides.

2. Step forward with the right foot keeping the left foot in place.

   Return to starting position and alternate legs.

Runs #9

REPS: 50x's

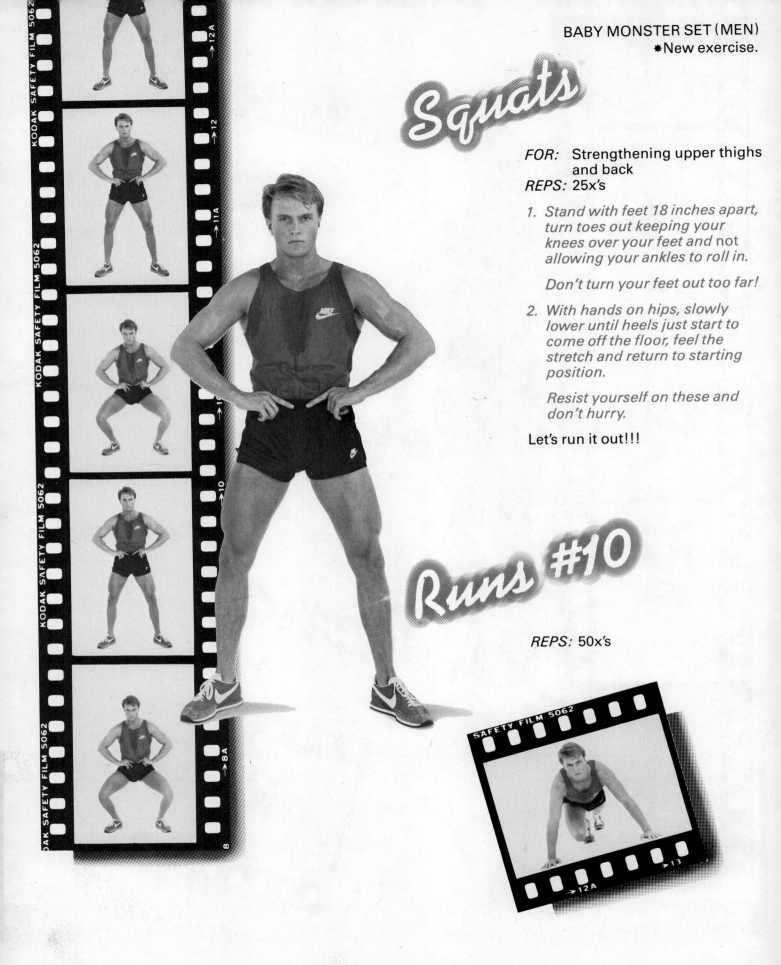

Squats

FOR: Strengthening upper thighs and back
REPS: 25x's

1. Stand with feet 18 inches apart, turn toes out keeping your knees over your feet and not allowing your ankles to roll in.

   Don't turn your feet out too far!

2. With hands on hips, slowly lower until heels just start to come off the floor, feel the stretch and return to starting position.

   Resist yourself on these and don't hurry.

   Let's run it out!!!

Runs #10

REPS: 50x's

Big Boy Push-Ups

REPS: Ladies: 5x's
Men: 25x's

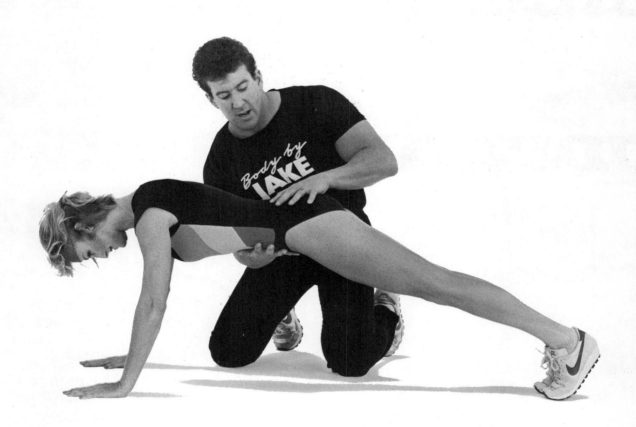

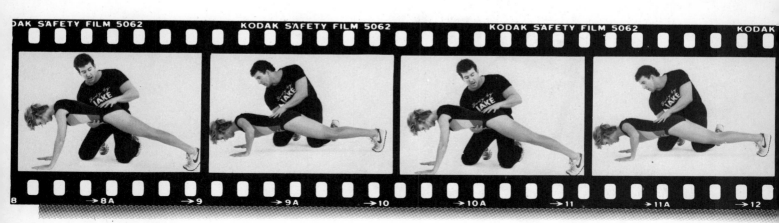

* Variation from previous chapter.

Leg Raises *

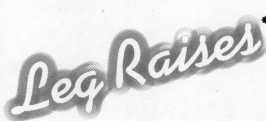

FOR: Stomach and thighs
REPS: 50x's for each set
TIME: 50 seconds for each set

These are all repeats from page 73. So get your hands under your "tushie" and your head raised with your chin on your chest and GO!

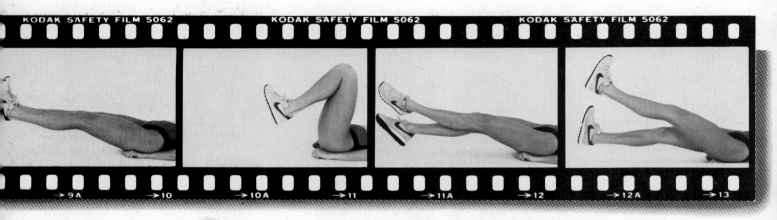

KODAK SAFETY FILM 5062 · KODAK SAFETY FILM 5062 · KODAK SAFETY FILM 5062

→9A →10 →10A →11 →11A →12 →12A →13

In/Outs

REPS: 50x's

Scissors

REPS: 50x's

Baby Runs

REPS: 50x's

DON'T EVER LET ME CATCH YOU WITH YOUR FEET NEAR THE FLOOR DURING THIS EXERCISE!!!

Aw right! It's time to get lean and mean for another 50 runs!

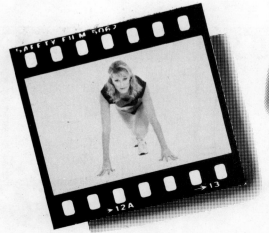

SAFETY FILM 5062

→12A →13

Runs #11

REPS: 50x's

Big Crunch ✱

FOR: Strengthening stomach and lower back
REPS: 50x's

1. Lie on back, raise head and shoulders about 6" from the floor.

2. Keeping knees straight raise feet off floor then bend one knee and try to touch it to opposite elbow. Alternating legs continue for full number of reps. Keep extended leg off the floor.

I want these fast, fast, fast!

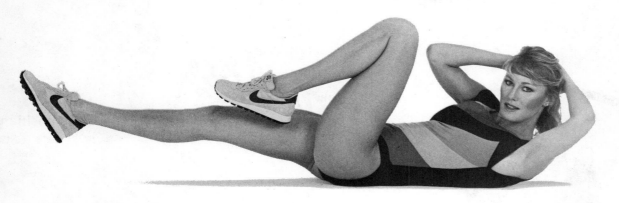

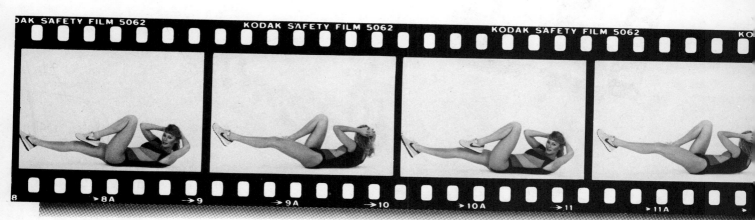

Wishbone Stretch

Almost through!!!!

Let's cool it down and stretch it out.

REPS: Hold for 25 in each position—left, right and center

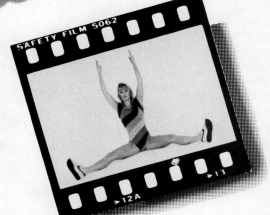

Hurdles

REPS: Hold for 25 in each position

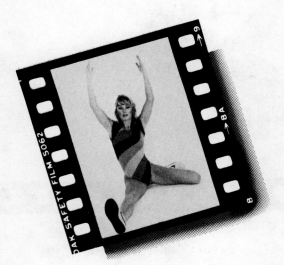

Eggroll

REPS: Hold until you're "rolled" out!

Go take a nice hot bath and read what I have to say about all this!

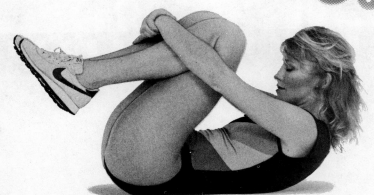

I bet you're really smoked now, huh? Well, if you want to burn calories besides get firm...this is how you have to do it!

There are a couple of other things you can do without working up such a sweat that will help out too.

Use your muscles to lift objects rather than push them.

Climb a few flights of stairs rather than using the elevator or escalator.

Put your arm straight out in front of you and push yourself away from the table.

Sit tall. Walk Tall. Remember, you're in the driver's seat and you don't have to buy a Rolls Royce to own a classy chassis!

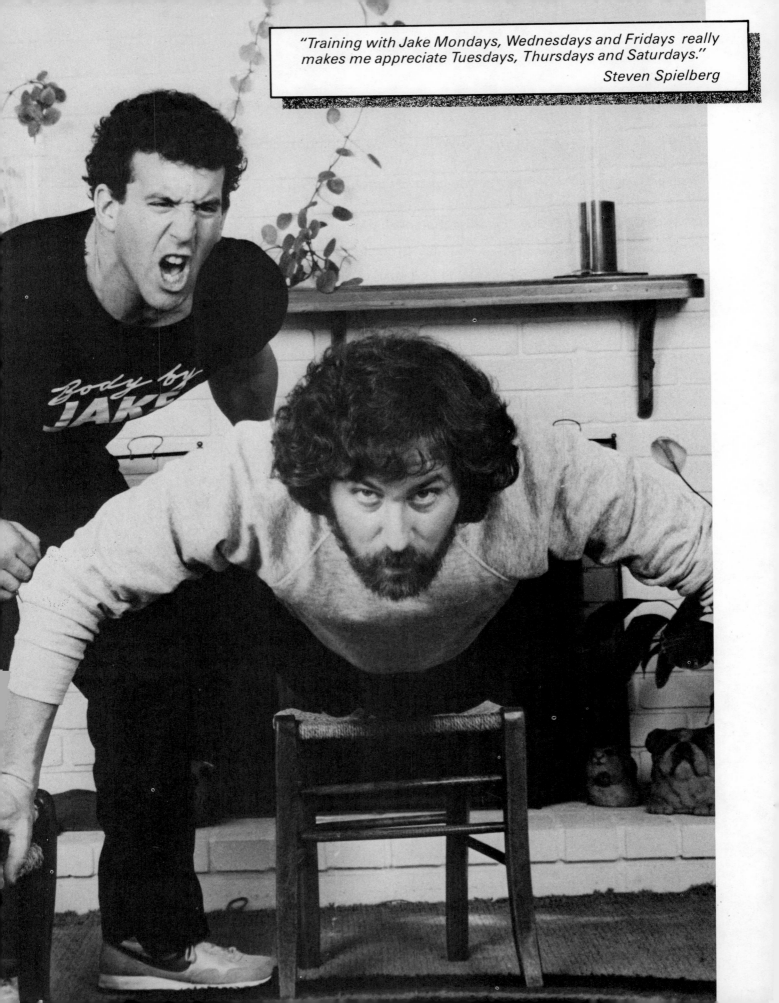

"Training with Jake Mondays, Wednesdays and Fridays really makes me appreciate Tuesdays, Thursdays and Saturdays."
Steven Spielberg

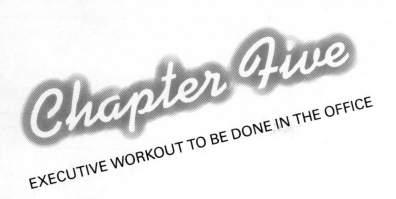

Chapter Five

EXECUTIVE WORKOUT TO BE DONE IN THE OFFICE

Hey! You know that funny feeling you get when things get crazy? It's called stress. It's your body responding to your brain. We all get it. It's our survival instinct that says... "fight or flight". And, whether you decide to stay and stick it out or, run away... your body gets ready in the same way. Your muscles tighten, your heart starts beating faster and there's that shot of adrenaline for energy. If you don't do anything with it, the feeling of stress stays and your body is still ready for "combat". Don't fight it! Use it!! Work it off!!!

Of course, the best way to take care of stress and tension is to be in good shape to begin with. If you've got good health, you've got a stronger and more efficient heart. You can take physical and emotional stress better. And, here's the best part, people in good shape have less nervous tension and are more mentally alert.

This Executive Workout doesn't require any special equipment. You can do it in your office, your kitchen or your bedroom depending on what kind of executive you are! You don't get wrinkled or sweaty! How long it takes is up to you. I've given you the chart with beginning reps and if you feel like increasing them... do it!

All these exercises are basically the ones you've learned throughout the book but modified for time, space and sweat. This program does not, I repeat, does not replace a truly smokin' Jake "The Snake" Workout with your "sweats" and "sneaks". What this program *can* do is relieve stress and/or get some oxygen into your body to help you through that mid-morning or mid-afternoon slump. It'll also let your body know you haven't forgotten about it! REMEMBER: do *not* do this workout if you haven't been working out with this book from page one! This is not one of those "drop in when you feel like it" exercise books!

So, get yourself a chair, some books and a wall and either sit in the corner and read something or move it around and get some energy.

EXECUTIVE WORKOUT

- TO BE DONE WHILE FULLY CLOTHED!
- REPETITIONS TO BE ADDED AT OWN DISCRETION
- THIS WORKOUT IS NOT TO REPLACE A "REAL" WORKOUT

CHAPTER FIVE

EXERCISES	Workout 1 REPS	Workout 1 U DID	Workout 2 REPS	Workout 2 U DID	Workout 3 REPS	Workout 3 U DID	Workout 4 REPS	Workout 4 U DID	Workout 5 REPS	Workout 5 U DID	GOAL
BIG STRETCH	10										
HEAD ROLLS	5										
*WHEEL ROLLS	15										
*PUSH-UPS OFF DESK	15										
*POWER PUSH	5	(HOLD FOR 5 COUNTS)									
*BIG SQUEEZE	5										
* SQUATS: SEMI	7										
FULL	15										
*CALF RAISES: ONE LEG	20										
TWO LEGS	20										
* IN CHAIR LEG RAISES	20										
* SCISSORS	20										
*BABY RUNS	20										
*LEG FREEZES	20	(HOLD FOR 20 COUNTS)									
*HANG LOOSE	5										

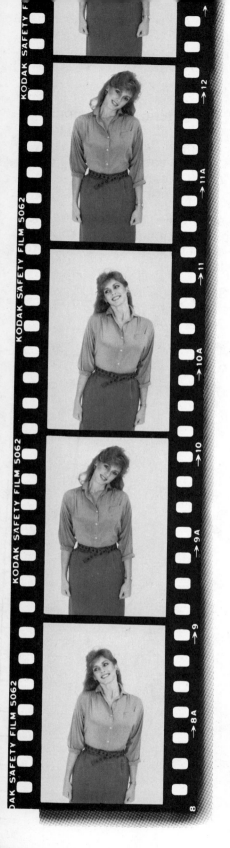

Big Stretch

REPS: 10x's

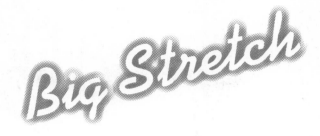

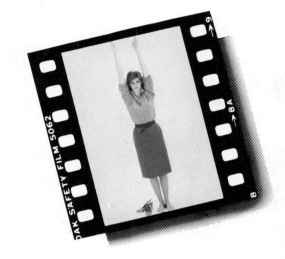

Head Rolls

REPS: 5x's each direction

Wheel Rolls

FOR: Warming up the upper body, strengthening the upper back.
REPS: 15x's each direction
TIME: 10 seconds in each direction

These are like arm circles but they won't make you sweat as much! We don't want you to "pit-out" that fresh shirt!

1. *Stand with arms out from shoulders like the old Arm Circles on page 19 .*

2. *Now swing the arms in GREAT BIG circles.*

   Gimme 15 WIDE circles in each direction!

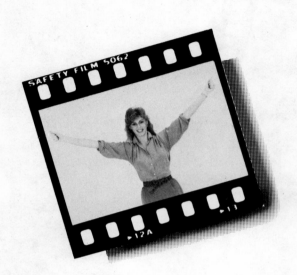

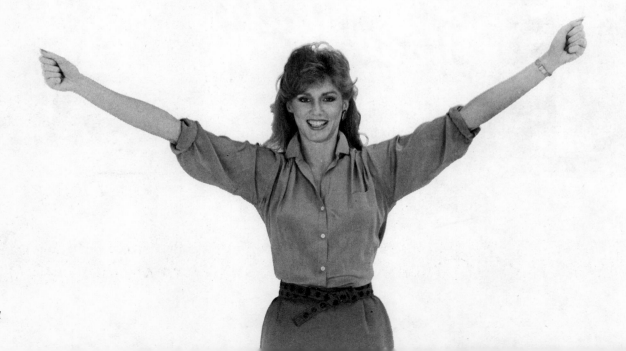

Push-Ups Off Desk

FOR: Toning and strengthening upper body and maintaining heart rate.
REPS: 15x's
TIME: 15 seconds

These will work the same as regular Push-ups without having to get down on the floor and get lint all over your navy blue suit.

1. Take the Push-up position with your toes on the floor and your hands shoulder width apart on the edge of a table or desk.

2. Raise and lower yourself like a regular Push-up with your chin touching the edge of the desk.

   Gimme 15 at a speed that won't make you sweat too much.

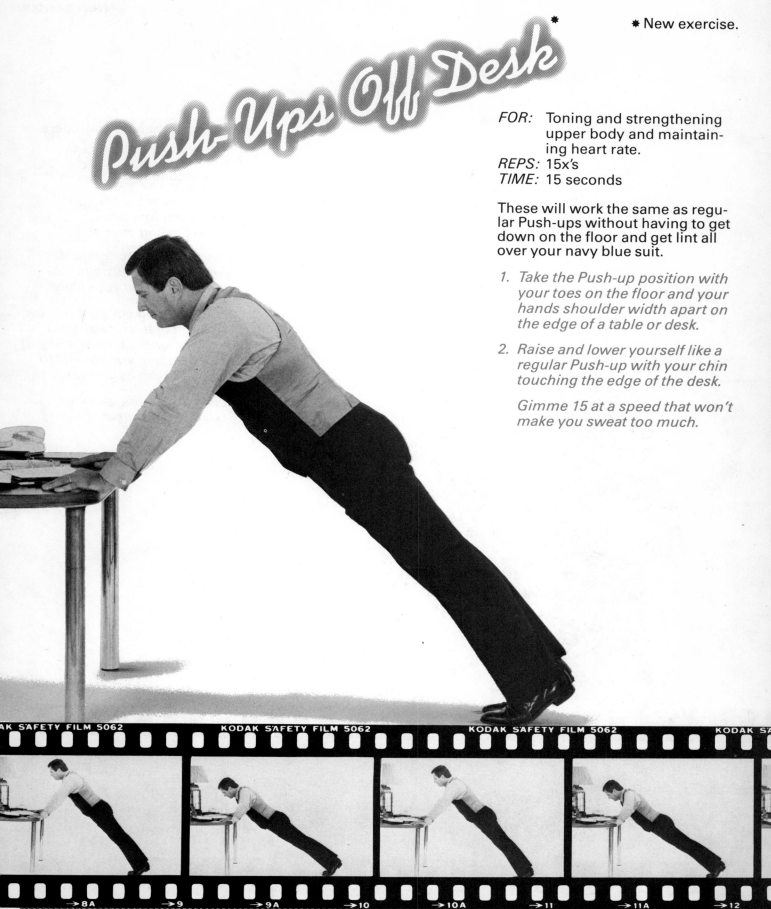

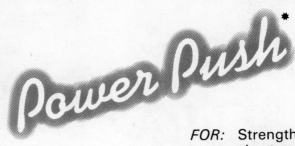

* New exercise.

Power Push

FOR: Strengthening shoulders, chest and arms.
REPS: 5x's
TIME: 5 seconds each

This isometric will work your shoulders and forearms without wrinkling your shirt!!!

1. *Standing with legs shoulder width apart, press palms together in front of your chest.*

2. *While resisting yourself (I know how hard that is!) push your arms straight out in front of you while pressing your palms together as hard as you can.*

   Return to starting position SLOWLY and repeat.

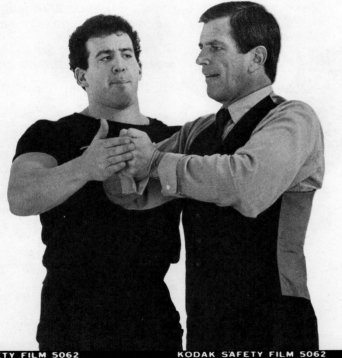

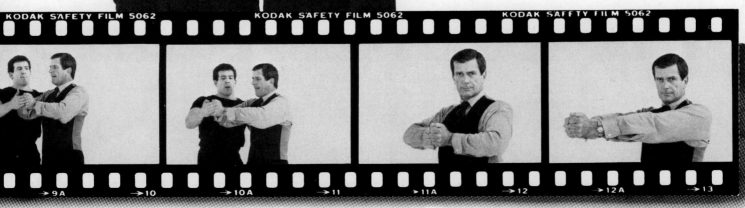

156

The Big Squeeze

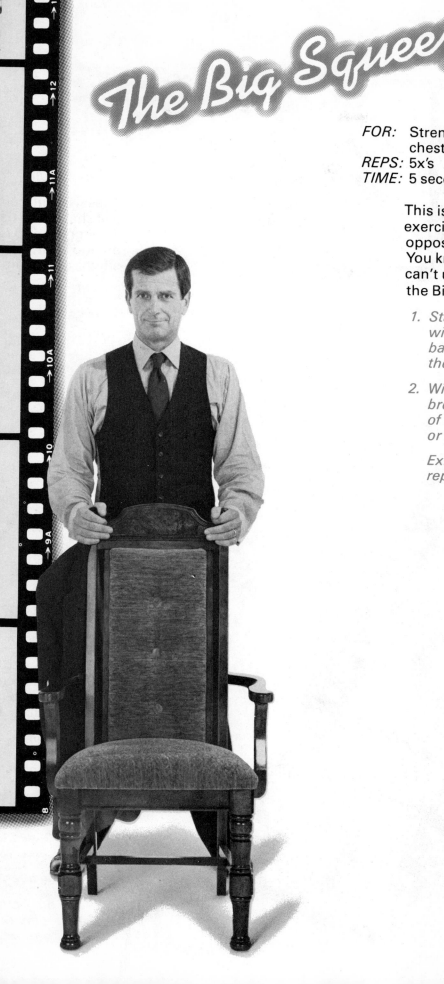

FOR: Strengthening shoulders, chest and arms.
REPS: 5x's
TIME: 5 seconds each

This is another isometric exercise but sorta the opposite of the Power Push. You know how it is ... if you can't use the Power Push try the Big Squeeze!!!

1. *Stand behind a chair with hands grasping the back of the chair from the sides, then inhale.*

2. *Without holding your breath squeeze the sides of the chair together... or at least try to.*

   Exhale, release and repeat.

157

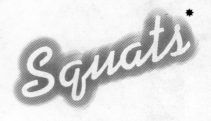

Squats ∗

REPS: 7 half
15 full

These are the same Squats as the last chapter on page *144* so gimme 7 halfers and 15 fulls. If your pants are too tight ... you can skip the full squats and gimme 21 halfers.

∗ New exercise.

Calf Raises ∗

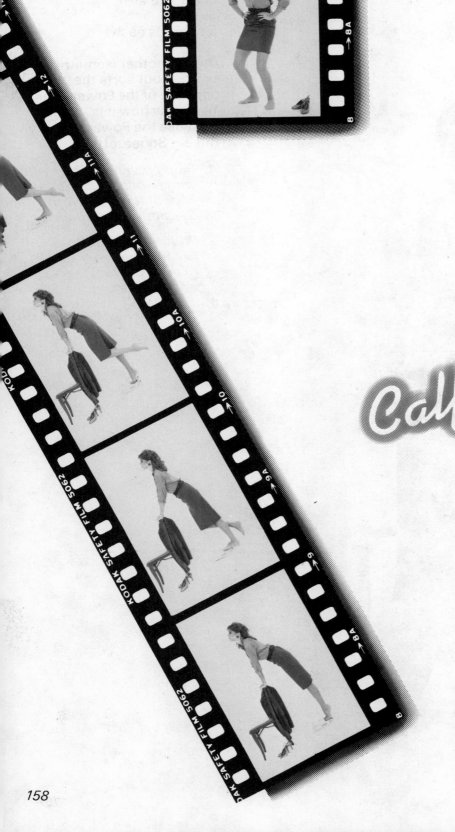

FOR: Calves!
REPS: 20x's single leg
20x's legs together
TIME: 20 seconds for 20x's

These are brand new to you so read the instructions carefully! You're going to need a stack of books about six inches high.

1. *Stand with the ball and arch of one foot on the stack of books and the heel off the edge.*

2. *Now rise up as high as you can on that foot.*

3. *Then lower as far below the books as you can.*

   Gimme twenty on each leg.

   Now put both feet on the books, and repeat the exercise for twenty more.

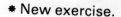

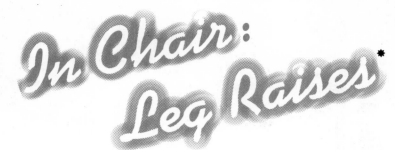

In Chair: Leg Raises *

FOR: Abdomens and upper thighs.
REPS: 20x's
TIME: 40 seconds

This is so much like regular leg raises that it'll be a cinch. The only difference is that you get to sit in a chair!

1. *Sit in chair with your legs extended in front and hold on to the sides of the chair.*

2. *Raise legs until they are level with the chair seat.*

3. *Now slowly lower to starting position and repeat.*

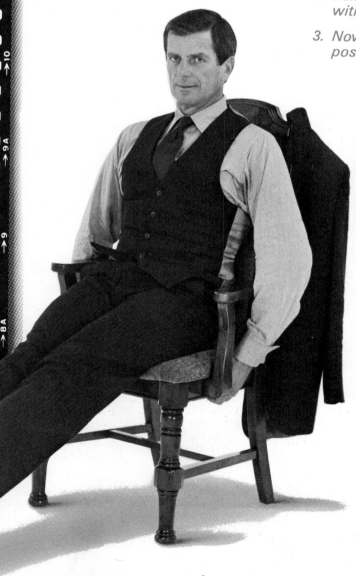

159

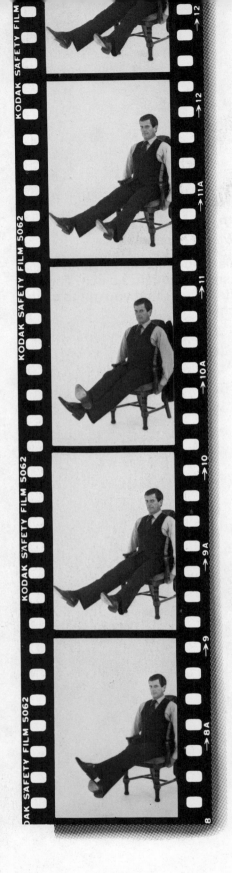

In Chair : Scissors *

REPS: 20x's

1. Sit in the chair like before with legs extended in front and hands gripping chair sides.

2. Raise legs to chair seat level and while holding them gimme twenty Scissors, crossing your legs back and forth.

Remember: don't sweat too much! And don't worry—we're almost through.

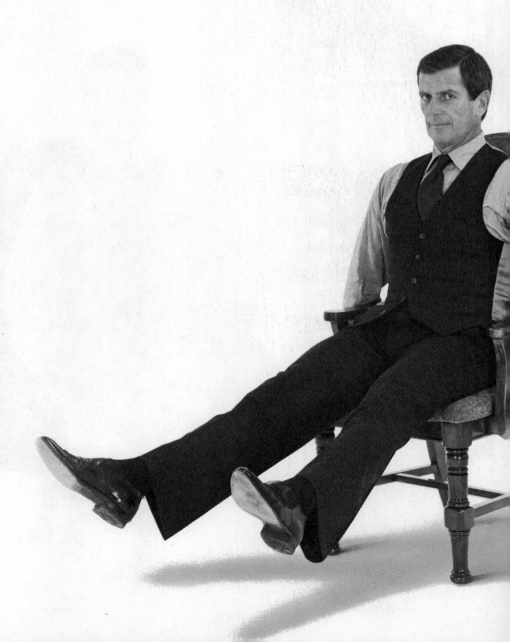

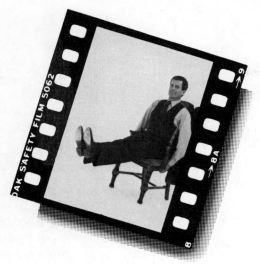

Baby Runs *

FOR: Abdomens and legs.
REPS: 20x's
TIME: 20 seconds

1. *Sit in the chair like before with legs extended in front and hands gripping chair sides.*

2. *Now do flexed foot Baby Runs just like you were doing Leg Raises on the floor.*

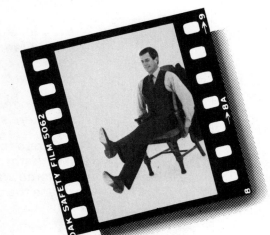

* New exercise.

Leg Freezes

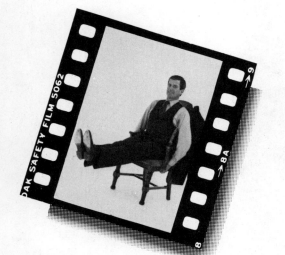

FOR: Abdomen and legs.
REPS: hold for 20 counts
TIME: 20 seconds

1. *Remain in the chair with legs extended and held at chair seat level, hold for twenty counts.*

That's it! Jump up and hang loose!

161

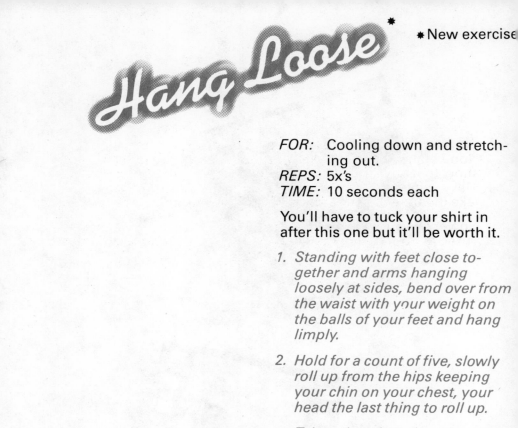

Hang Loose*

FOR: Cooling down and stretch-
ing out.
REPS: 5x's
TIME: 10 seconds each

You'll have to tuck your shirt in
after this one but it'll be worth it.

1. *Standing with feet close together and arms hanging
loosely at sides, bend over from
the waist with your weight on
the balls of your feet and hang
limply.*

2. *Hold for a count of five, slowly
roll up from the hips keeping
your chin on your chest, your
head the last thing to roll up.*

   *Take a deep breath and repeat
the exercise.*

Now, go to the rest room, kitchen
sink or bathroom, splash your face
with some water, tuck your shirt in,
and face the world.

So, how was it? Feel revitalized? Did you sweat too much? Did you rip the seat of your pants out? None of the above? I guarantee that once you're familiar with this routine you'll be hooked. Tests show that any kind of exercise helps to ease stress and the best ones are repetitive and rhythmic. Maybe that's why people count to ten over and over again. But I figure as long as you're gonna take the time to count to ten you might as well get some exercise.

Now make sure your next workout is in "sweats" and "sneaks" and you're back in Chapter Two, Three or Four giving me a full blown, smokin' workout! This isn't a substitute program! It's additional!

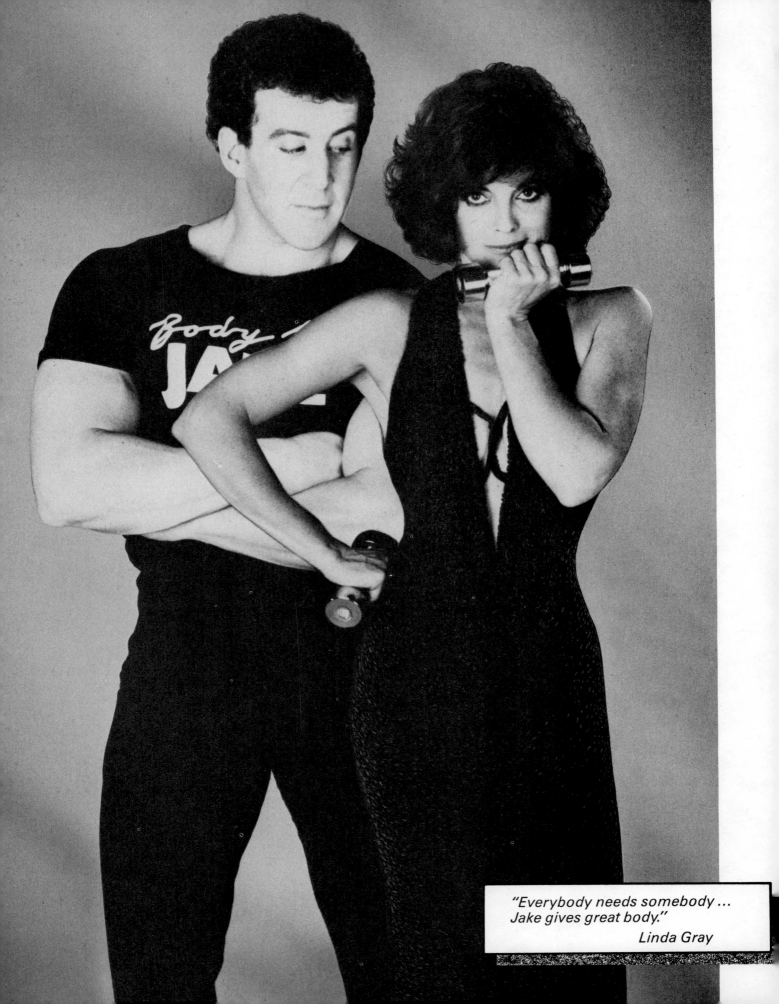

*"Everybody needs somebody ...
Jake gives great body."*
Linda Gray

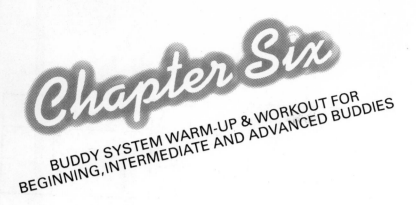

Chapter Six

BUDDY SYSTEM WARM-UP & WORKOUT FOR BEGINNING, INTERMEDIATE AND ADVANCED BUDDIES

I've been working out for years now and because I use very heavy weights I've always had a training partner. And, you know what? The few times I've had to exercise alone, when I've been on the road, it wasn't as much fun. And that's what this chapter is all about. Why do it alone if there's somebody around to do it with?

It's the old Buddy System. Just like in grammar school only now *you* get to choose the buddy. And a little healthy competition never hurt anyone. But that's not the only reason to exercise once in a while with someone else. Maybe you've been working out for a while and hit a slump. Maybe you need a break from the Baby Monster Set. Don't get bored when you workout. Just get a buddy. A buddy'll give you some encouragement and that little push you need to keep going. And you know, maybe you can do the same for somebody else. Maybe someone you care about needs some exercise and can't get started. Start together. Talk about goals. Schedule to workout together for a while. It'll be nice. Of course, like I said earlier, any of you who have gone on to heavier weights know that you have no choice. It's a basic safety rule. If you don't have a buddy to spot you . . . you don't work out!

Besides being physically healthy, working out with a buddy *could* be socially healthy too . . . if you don't choose your old buddy from grammar school. There are just a couple of things you have to consider before and after you get a buddy. Everybody is different. Not everybody is in the same physical condition. Be careful you're not making anyone do anything that is too difficult. And, be sure you don't hurt yourself either. This chapter is broken up for beginner, intermediate and advanced. If your partner hasn't followed my training program before, start him or her at a beginner level. You can start at the same level you are working at in Chapter One, Two, Three or Four. I assume that one of you is very familiar with my program! Otherwise your workout will be the blind leading the blind and then the injured leading the injured! One of you MUST be familiar with the exercises!

You're gonna need two broomsticks, two towels and twice as much room.

So, go get a buddy. You don't always have to be your own best friend when you exercise!

· MAKE SURE *BOTH* PARTNERS ARE FAMILIAR
WITH THE EXERCISES—AVOID INJURY!!!

CHAPTER SIX

EXERCISES	BEGINNER				INTERMEDIATE				ADVANCED		
	REPS	U DID	REPS	U DID	REPS	U DID	REPS	U DID	REPS	U DID	
BIG STRETCH	3				5				10		
HEAD ROLLS	3				5				5		
*BENT OVER ARM CIRCLES	30				35				50		
*BENT OVER PULLS	15				20				30		
BROOMSTICK: SIDE STRETCHES	15				20				30		
SINGLE SIDE STRETCHES	15				20				30		
TOE TOUCHES	15				20				50		
RUNS #1	15				20				50		
*RESISTER BUTT BURNERS	10				20				25		
PUSH-UPS (all)	5				10				25		
RUNS #2	15				20				50		
*RESISTER INNER THIGH (Women)	10				20				25		
*RESISTER SQUATS	5				10				15		
*RESISTER SIT-UPS	15				20				30		
LEG RAISES—IN/OUT	15				20				25		
SCISSORS	15				20				25		
BABY RUNS	15				20				25		
RUNS #3	15				20				50		

EXERCISES	BEGINNER				INTERMEDIATE				ADVANCED		
	REPS	U DID	REPS	U DID	REPS	U DID	REPS	U DID	REPS	U DID	
RESISTER BUTT BURNERS (Women)	10				20				25		
PUSH-UPS (all)	5				10				25		
*TOWEL PULLS	10				12				15		
*TOWEL CURLS	10				12				15		
*TOWEL TRIMENS	10				12				15		
RESISTER INNER THIGH (Women)	10				20				25		
RUNS #4	15				20				50		
LUNGES	10				15				25		
*RESISTER WISHBONE STRETCH	1	(10 COUNTS)			1	(15 COUNTS)			1	(25 COUNTS)	
HURDLES	1	(10 COUNTS)			1	(15 COUNTS)			1	(25 COUNTS)	

Big Stretch

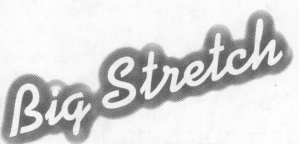

REPS: each side

BEGINNER	INTERMEDIATE	ADVANCED
3x's	5x's	10x's

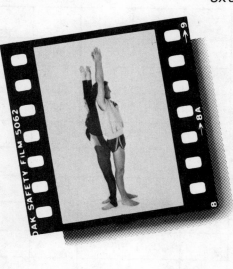

Head Rolls

REPS: each direction

3x's	5x's	5x's

Bent Over Arm Circles

REPS: each direction

BEGINNER   *INTERMEDIATE*   *ADVANCED*

30x's   35x's   50x's

These are the same arm circles
BUT....

1. *Bent over from the waist with knees slightly bent and proceed with arm circles as on page 123.*

Bent Over Pulls

FOR: Strengthening back, shoulders, and arms.

REPS: hold

15 counts   20 counts   30 counts

1. *Begin by 'facing' one another, grasping crossed hands and with knees bent.*

2. *Sit back on your heels and feel the pull in your arms.*

   If you like your partner a whole bunch, let his/her pull be strong enough to pull you towards 'em!

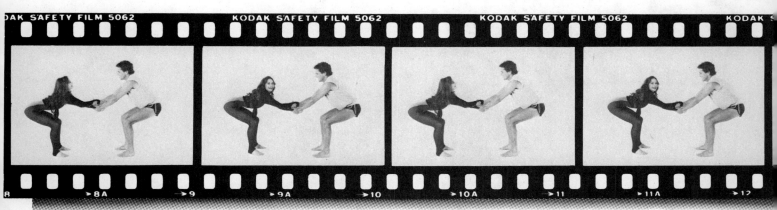

KODAK SAFETY FILM 5062

8A →9 →9A →10 →10A →11 →11A →12

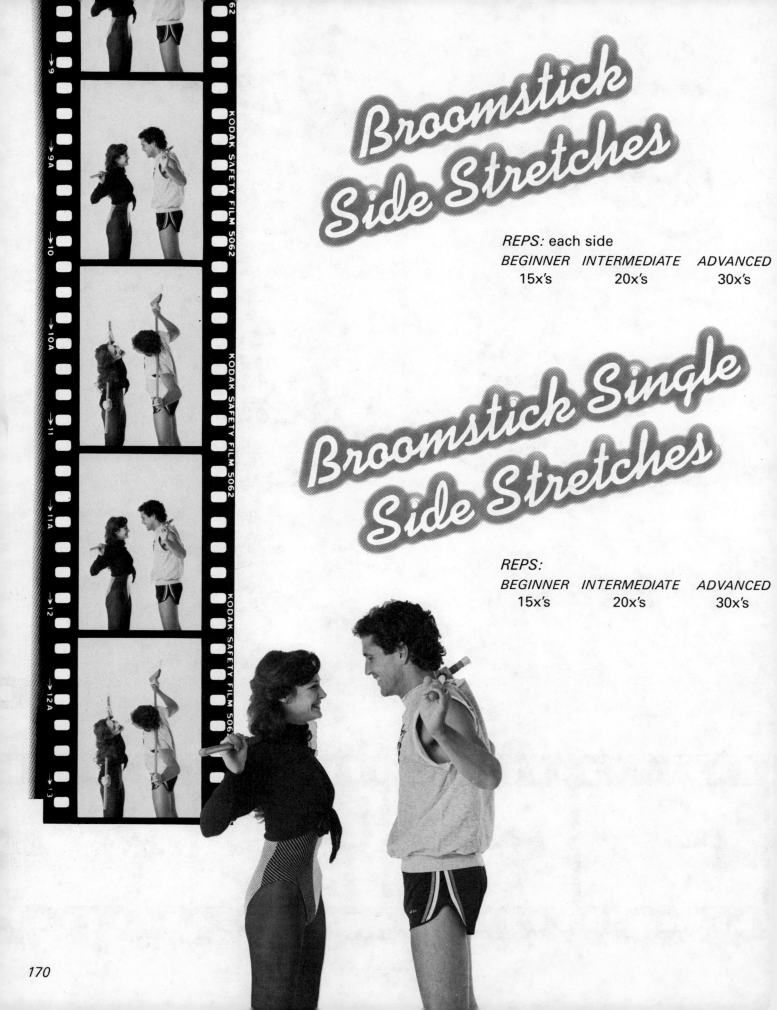

Broomstick Side Stretches

REPS: each side

BEGINNER	INTERMEDIATE	ADVANCED
15x's	20x's	30x's

Broomstick Single Side Stretches

REPS:

BEGINNER	INTERMEDIATE	ADVANCED
15x's	20x's	30x's

Toe Touches

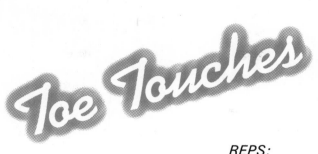

REPS:

BEGINNER	INTERMEDIATE	ADVANCED
15x's	20x's	50x's

Hips and up, hips and down...touching your own hips!

Runs #1

REPS:

BEGINNER	INTERMEDIATE	ADVANCED
15x's	20x's	50x's

Now we're gonna get down and get together.

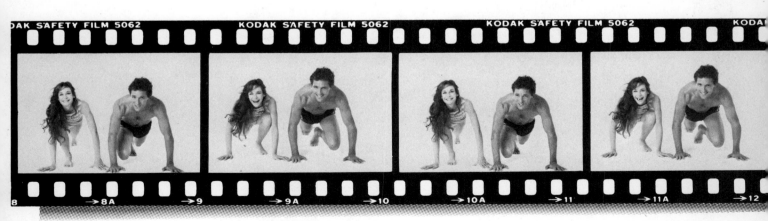

Resister Butt Burners

REPS: each leg

BEGINNER	INTERMEDIATE	ADVANCED
10x's	20x's	25x's

These are just like the other Butt Burners but now your partner will help you resist.

Remember: If you're exerting pressure on someone for a resiste don't exert so much pressure that they're defeated! The resistance i just to make it harder... not impossible.

1. *On hands and knees with leg extended straight out in the back as on page 66.*

   Partner holds one hand over c of the extended leg so that wh you raise it you can only go s far.

2. *Push your leg against the han as hard as possible trying to g it higher.*

   Return to starting position an repeat.

Pretty hard huh? You were at the advanced workout before you started this chapter? Better go bac to the Intermediate Reps!

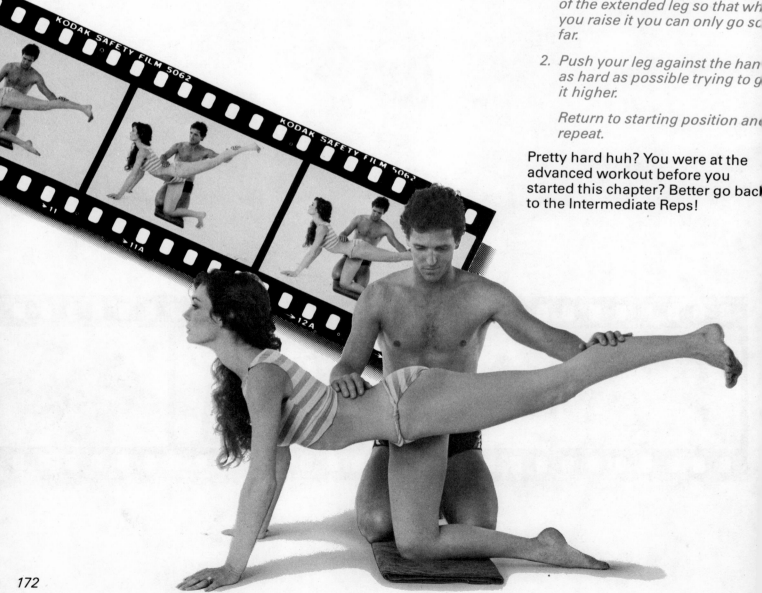

172

Big Boy Push-Ups

AND/OR

(WOMEN)

Knee Push-Ups

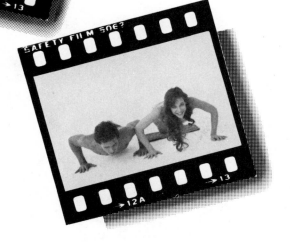

REPS:

BEGINNER	INTERMEDIATE	ADVANCED
5x's	10x's	25x's

You know how to do these Push-ups by now.

Lead with your chest and not with your chin! No matter if you're on your knees or straight out.

Both of you stay down there now for some runs!

Runs #2

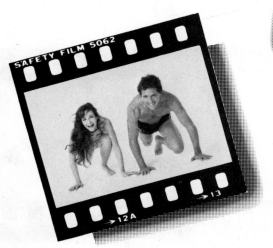

REPS:

BEGINNER	INTERMEDIATE	ADVANCED
15x's	20x's	50x's

Time for more resisters.

Ladies!

173

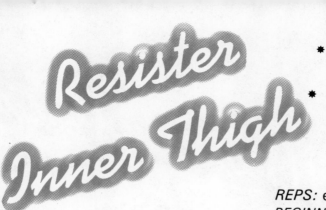

Resister Inner Thigh

REPS: each leg

BEGINNER	INTERMEDIATE	ADVANCED
10x's	20x's	25x's

These are the same as the beginning inner thigh work with the difference being the PARTNER PUSHING ON THE WORKING LEG.

1. On your side with top leg bent over bottom, your hand grasping your ankle.

2. Lift bottom leg up and push against partner's hand which he has placed on the ankle of the extended leg.

   Do not allow working leg to return to floor but complete all reps at once.

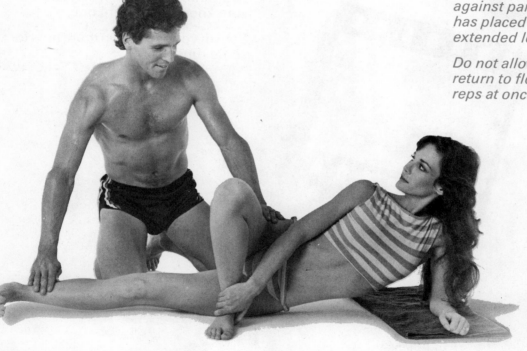

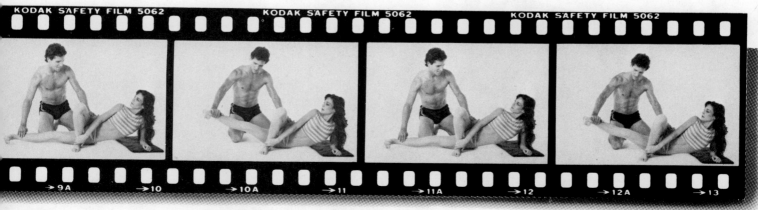

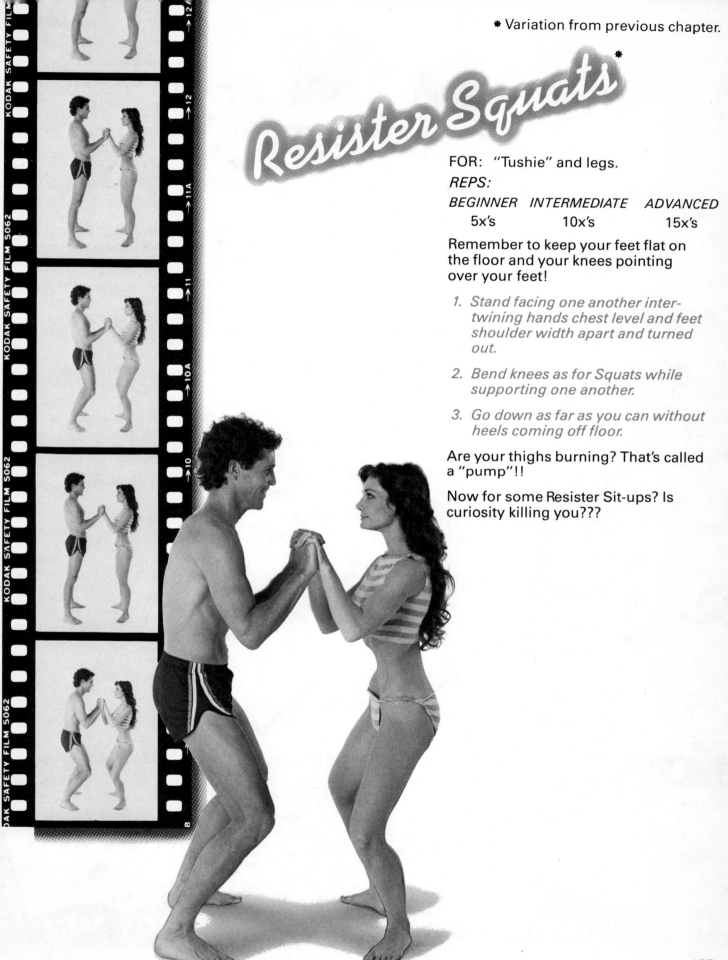

Resister Squats ✱

FOR: "Tushie" and legs.

REPS:

BEGINNER	*INTERMEDIATE*	*ADVANCED*
5x's	10x's	15x's

Remember to keep your feet flat on the floor and your knees pointing over your feet!

1. *Stand facing one another intertwining hands chest level and feet shoulder width apart and turned out.*

2. *Bend knees as for Squats while supporting one another.*

3. *Go down as far as you can without heels coming off floor.*

Are your thighs burning? That's called a "pump"!!

Now for some Resister Sit-ups? Is curiosity killing you???

Resister Double Sit-Ups *

REPS:

BEGINNER	INTERMEDIATE	ADVANCED
15x's	20x's	30x's

These are a special kind of bent knee Sit-ups here. You'll see why after you do them.

1. Sit facing one another with feet locked around each other by one person putting legs under as the partner has her's over.

2. Proceed as for "Big Crunch" on page 147, touching elbow to opposite knee, returning to start position and alternating opposite elbow to opposite knee.

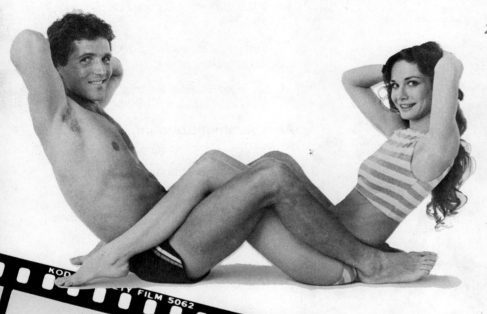

Leg Raises

These are the same Leg Raises as the first chapter. Hands under "tushie," fists clenched, head held up, legs straight out and never touching the floor! Now go for it together!

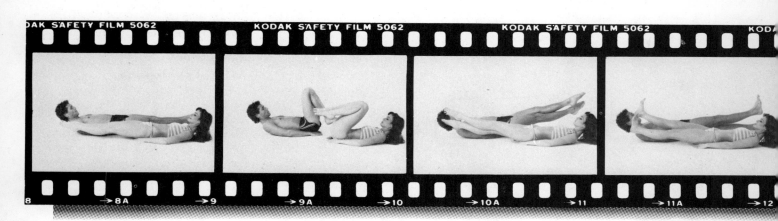

In/Outs
Scissors
Baby Runs

REPS:		
BEGINNER	INTERMEDIATE	ADVANCED
15x's	20x's	25x's
15x's	20x's	25x's
15x's	20x's	25x's

Runs #3

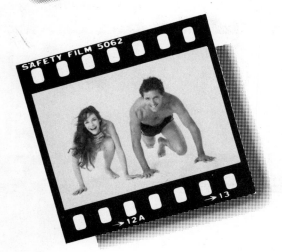

REPS:		
BEGINNER	INTERMEDIATE	ADVANCED
15x's	20x's	50x's

Get ready to resist again.

We're gonna repeat a whole set of Burners, Push-ups and something new!

Resister Butt Burners

REPS: each side

BEGINNER	INTERMEDIATE	ADVANCED
10x's	20x's	25x's

I know it's tough but keep resisting!

1. On hands and knees, extend one leg straight out in the back.

   Partner holds one hand over ankle of extended leg so that when you raise it you can only go so far.

2. Push your leg against the hand as hard as possible trying to get it higher each time.

   Return to starting position and repeat.

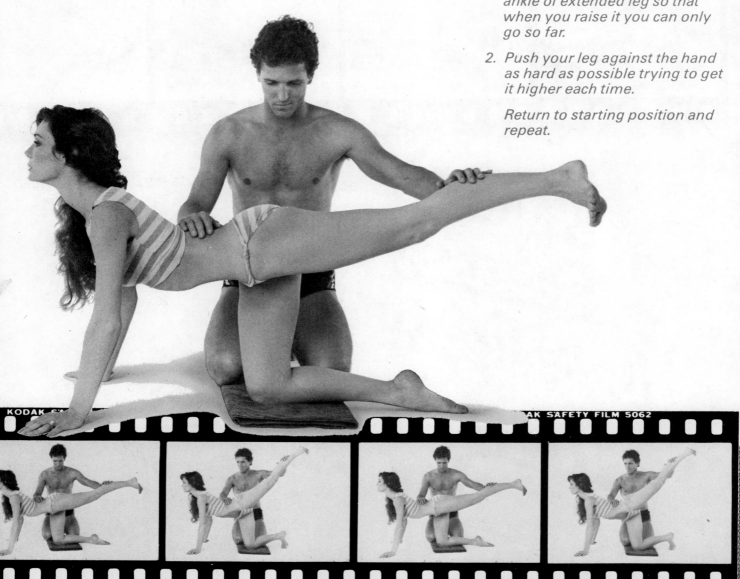

178

Big Boy Push-Ups

OR

Knee Push-Ups

REPS:

BEGINNER	INTERMEDIATE	ADVANCED
5x's	10x's	25x's

It's now time to resist your upper body! Hope you have a good partner!

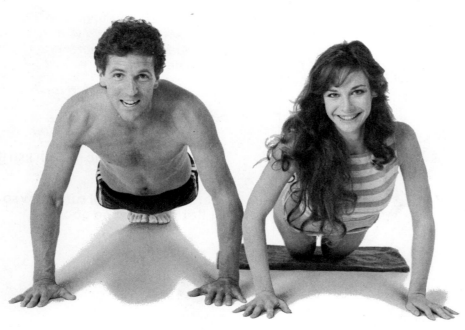

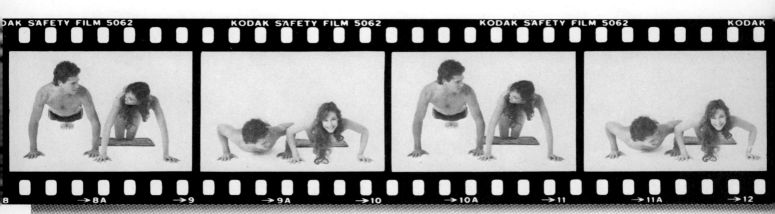

Towel Pulls *

FOR: Strengthening back and arms.
REPS:

BEGINNER	INTERMEDIATE	ADVANCED
10x's	12x's	15x's

Towel pulls are like when you used to play with your dog and an old sock. He'd grab the sock in his mouth and he'd pull one end and you'd pull the other.

Now you're gonna use a towel, you and your partner are gonna be at either end of it and, hopefully your partner is *not* a dog!

1. *Each of you take one end of the towel and hold it taut between you with one partner sitting and one bending over.*

2. *Both pull back and forth alternating resistance.*

   Hold for 10, 12 or 15 counts.

Feels pretty good to stretch like that huh?

Let's do some towel curls now so it'll stop feeling so good.

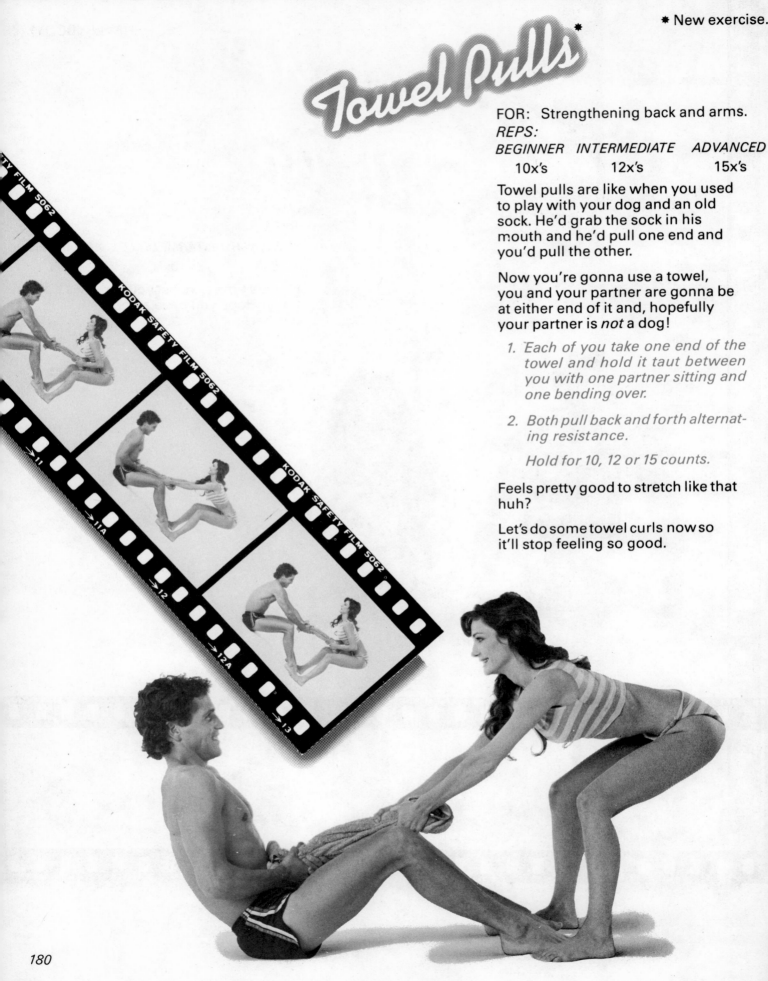

Resister Inner Thighs

REPS:

BEGINNER	INTERMEDIATE	ADVANCED
10x's	20x's	25x's

Do it just the same as before.

1. *On your side with top leg bent over bottom, hand grasping ankle.*

2. *Lift leg up and push against partner's hand.*

   Do not allow working leg to return to floor but complete all reps at once.

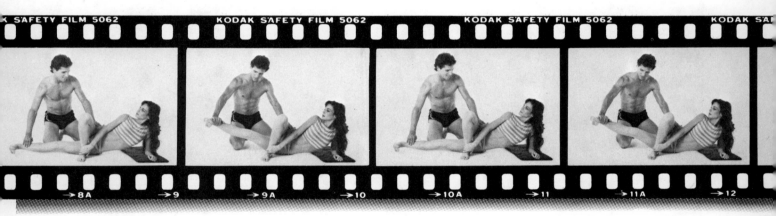

Runs #4

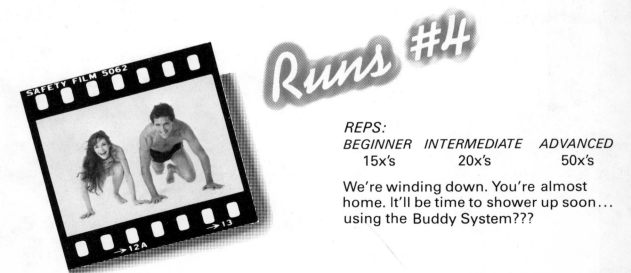

REPS:

BEGINNER	INTERMEDIATE	ADVANCED
15x's	20x's	50x's

We're winding down. You're almost home. It'll be time to shower up soon... using the Buddy System???

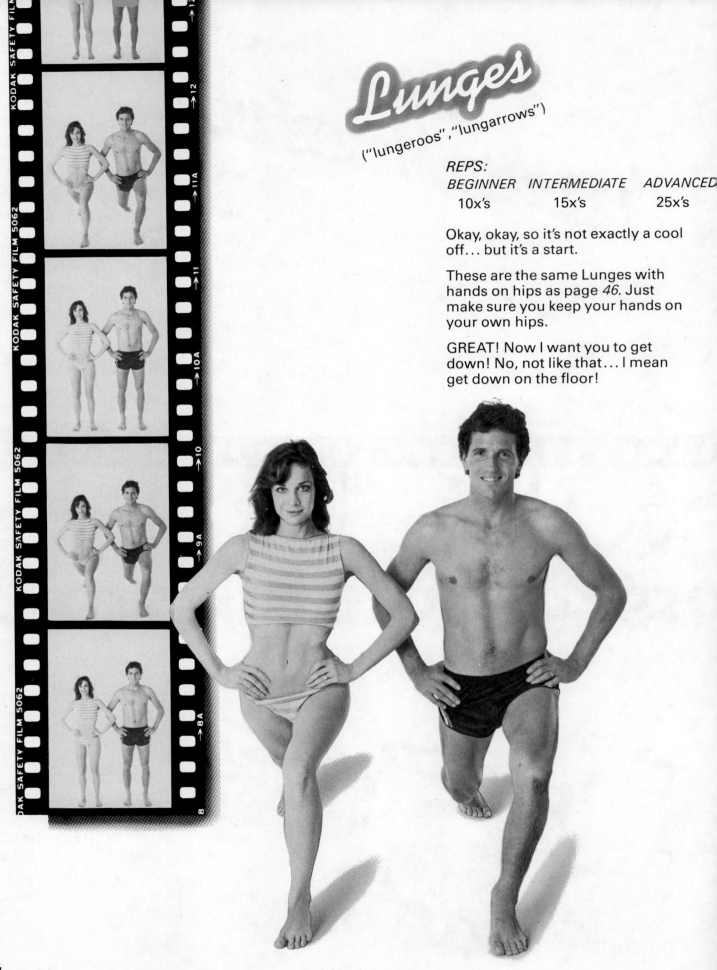

Lunges
("lungeroos","lungarrows")

REPS:
BEGINNER	INTERMEDIATE	ADVANCED
10x's	15x's	25x's

Okay, okay, so it's not exactly a cool off... but it's a start.

These are the same Lunges with hands on hips as page *46*. Just make sure you keep your hands on your own hips.

GREAT! Now I want you to get down! No, not like that... I mean get down on the floor!

Resister Wishbone Stretches *

REPS:

BEGINNER	INTERMEDIATE	ADVANCED
1	1	1
(10 counts)	(15 counts)	(25 counts)

This is just like the wishbone stretch you've always done to cool down only now... HARDER.

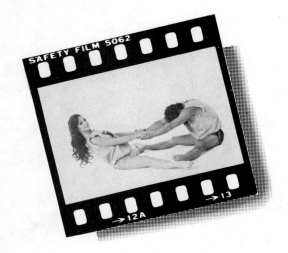

1. Sit facing your partner, both of you with legs in wishbone stretch position.

   One of you should put your feet on the other's inner ankle as the two of you grasp each others wrists and gently pull one another back and forth holding for the recommended number of counts.

2. Now reverse positions with the other person having his or her feet on your inner ankle.

   Again slowly rock back and forth.

Extra-Stretch Hurdles

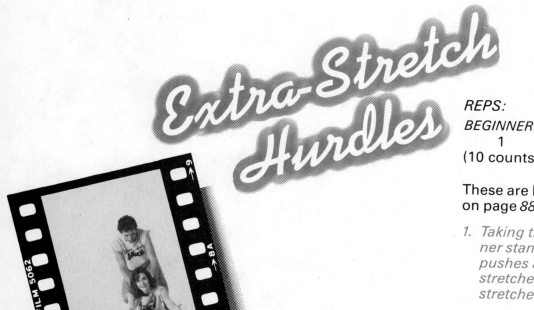

REPS:

BEGINNER	INTERMEDIATE	ADVANCED
1	1	1
(10 counts)	(15 counts)	(25 counts)

These are like the regular Hurdles on page 88 only....

1. Taking the hurdle position, partner stands behind and gently pushes as the "hurdler" stretches forward over outstretched leg.

2. Change legs.

   Reverse positions.

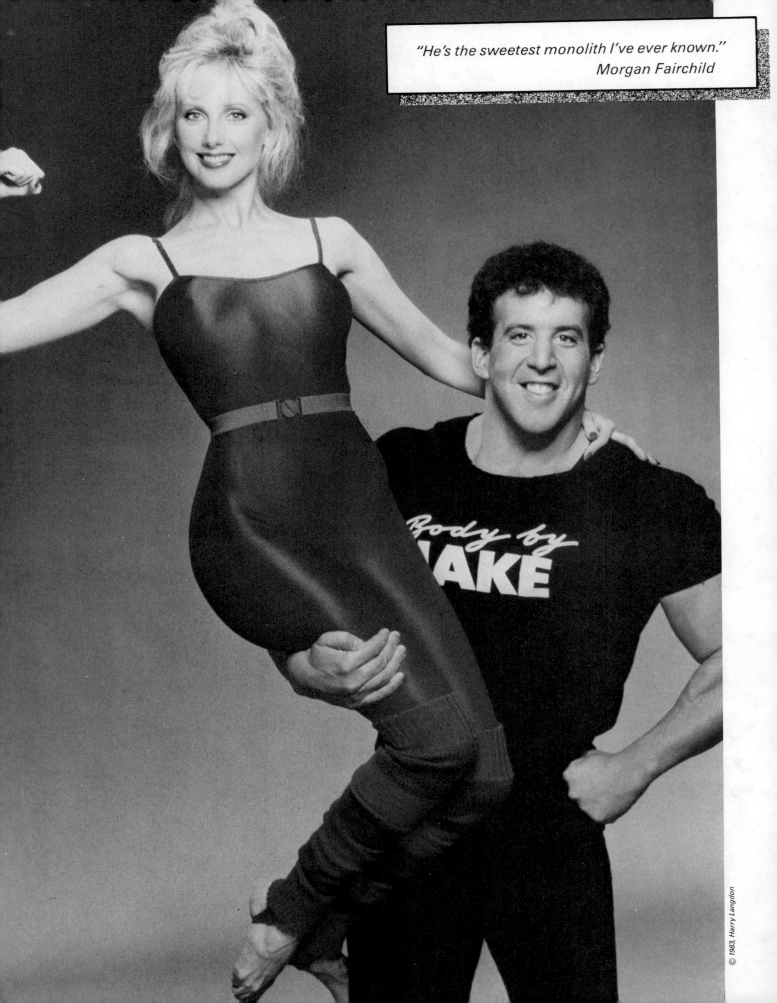

"He's the sweetest monolith I've ever known."
Morgan Fairchild

© 1983, Harry Langdon

Well, how was it? Did you take a shower afterwards? Go out for some sushi? Elope to Las Vegas and start a family? Or wasn't this that kind of a buddy. Let me ask you this then; how was the workout? Were the stretches tougher and the resisters harder? I told you so! It's good for you. I'm telling you exercise never has to be boring! As long as you stick with "The Snake" here we're always gonna have a good workout!

What do you say we take it on the road now?

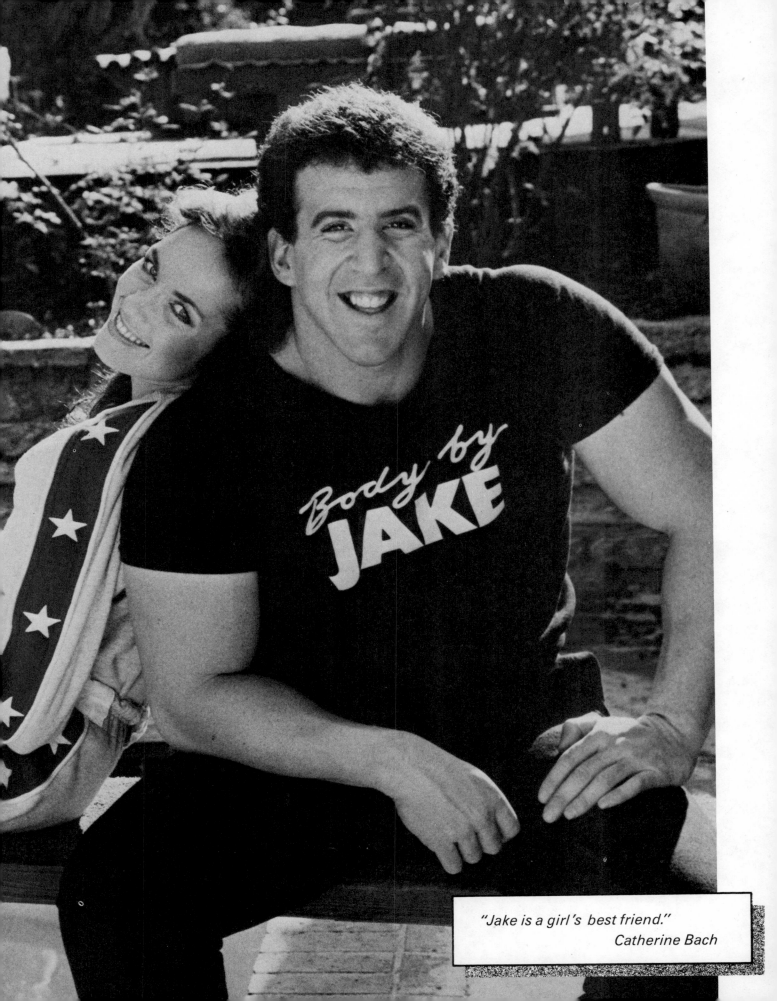

"Jake is a girl's best friend."
Catherine Bach

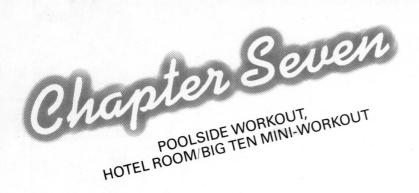

Chapter Seven

POOLSIDE WORKOUT, HOTEL ROOM/BIG TEN MINI-WORKOUT

Gee, here we are alone in a hotel room together. I guess after all the workouts we've had together, this should be easy…

How about, before we get into anything here, how about if we talk a little bit first? I mean, you know, we've always had a little "schmooze" before we've started work. Let's talk about what we've already done and maybe what we're gonna do.

Let's see. You got your beginning warm-up and workout in Chapter One. That took two weeks. Then you got your regular warm-up and workout with variations in Chapter Two. I guess that's where we really started to understand each other 'cause the next thing you knew we started to get heavy. I introduced you to some free weights. (Who says nothing is free in this life?) The next thing you knew, I got personal. I talked to you about your fat! I thought you took it real well. That's when I had you do the Baby Monster Set. I know that I really smoked some of you in the beginning with that Set but it had to happen!

Next thing you knew I made you take me to work with you!!! I had to go. I can't have my clients running around with their bodies pumpin' on STRESS! So you learned an extra workout for those special occasions. Next we worked out with buddies. And you know how I feel about that: "Why do it alone if there's somebody around to do it with?" And now, here we are alone in a hotel room.

I guess you thought if you left home you could leave your workout. No way. Where there's a will there's a workout no matter where you are. We do have two choices on this one though. You can workout in the hotel pool for a nice variation and don't worry. You're not gonna look dumb. It's underwater. And, if it's too cold or your bathing suit shrunk, I got The Big Ten Mini-Workout for you. But let me tell you something one more time. Neither one of these workouts is a substitute for a real Jake "The Snake" Workout that is a full-blown smokin' half-hour. These workouts are for those times that you don't have your equipment or the time *but* they're not for "at home"! At home you gotta do the full workout.

There are very few explanations for these workouts.

If you don't know the exercises then you have no business trying this workout and you should have bought the book yourself and not borrowed your friend's and you should start at the beginning and learn the program the right way and you probably didn't check with your doctor first either!

So, let's get out of this room and into the pool. Or, you can change into something comfortable for the best ten minutes you've ever had in a hotel room.

• ADD REPETITIONS AT OWN DISCRETION

CHAPTER SEVEN

EXERCISES	Workout 1 REPS	Workout 1 UDID	Workout 2 REPS	Workout 2 UDID	Workout 3 REPS	Workout 3 UDID	Workout 4 REPS	Workout 4 UDID	Workout 5 REPS	Workout 5 UDID	GOAL
BIG STRETCH	10										
HEAD ROLLS	5										
ARM CIRCLES	50										
TWISTERS	50										
*SIDE: STRETCHES	20										
SINGLE STRETCHES	20										
OVER HEAD	20										
SINGLE OVER HEAD	20										
TOE TOUCHES	35										
RUNS	50										
FROG KICKS #1	15										
ELBOW RUNS #1	15										
TOWEL PULLS	3	(HOLD FOR 15 COUNTS)									
*POOL PUSH-UPS	15										
*POOL LADDER PUSH-UPS	15										
*POOL EDGE PUSH-UPS	15										
*POOL LADDER DIPS	15										
INVERTED CURL PULL-UPS	15										
DIVING BOARD PULL-UPS	10										
*TREADING WATER WITH ARM SWINGS	20										

HOTEL ROOM WORKOUT/BIG 10 MINI-WORKOUT

EXERCISES	Workout 1 REPS	Workout 1 U DID	Workout 2 REPS	Workout 2 U DID	Workout 3 REPS	Workout 3 U DID	Workout 4 REPS	Workout 4 U DID	Workout 5 REPS	Workout 5 U DID	GOAL
10 HEAD ROLLS	5										
10 ARM CIRCLES	10										
10 WHEEL ROLLS	10										
10 TWISTERS	10										
10 SIDE STRETCHES	10										
10 SINGLE SIDE STRETCHES	10										
10 OVER HEAD SIDE STRETCHES	10										
10 COUNT SINGLE OVER HEAD	1		(HOLD FOR 10 COUNTS)								
10 TOE TOUCHES	10										
10 RUNS	10										
10 BODY BURNERS	10										
10 RUNS	10										
10 PUSH-UPS OFF BED	10										
10 RUNS	10										
10 SIT-UPS/FEET UNDER BED	10										
10 RUNS	10										
10 LEG RAISES	10										
IN/OUTS	10										
SCISSORS	10										
BABY RUNS	20										
10 COUNT WISHBONE STRETCH	10										
10 COUNT HURDLES	10										

191

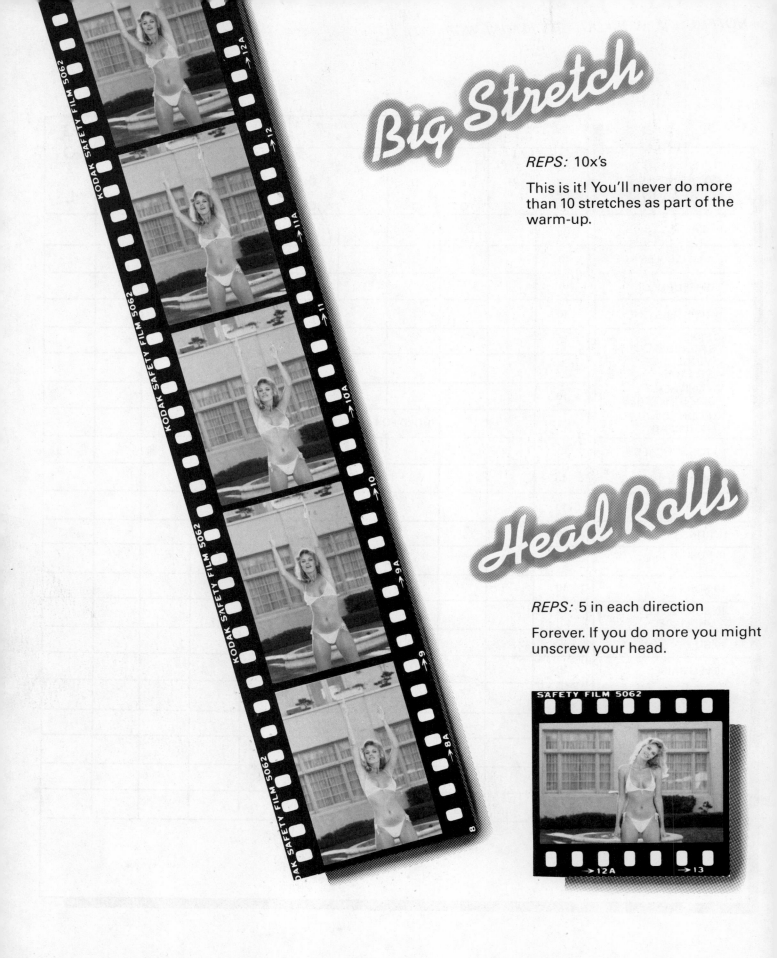

Big Stretch

REPS: 10x's

This is it! You'll never do more than 10 stretches as part of the warm-up.

Head Rolls

REPS: 5 in each direction

Forever. If you do more you might unscrew your head.

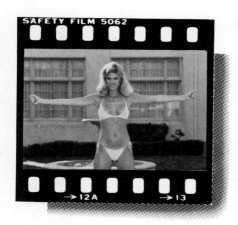

Arm Circles

REPS: 50 in each direction
Never more, never less.

Twisters

REPS: 50
Ultimate.

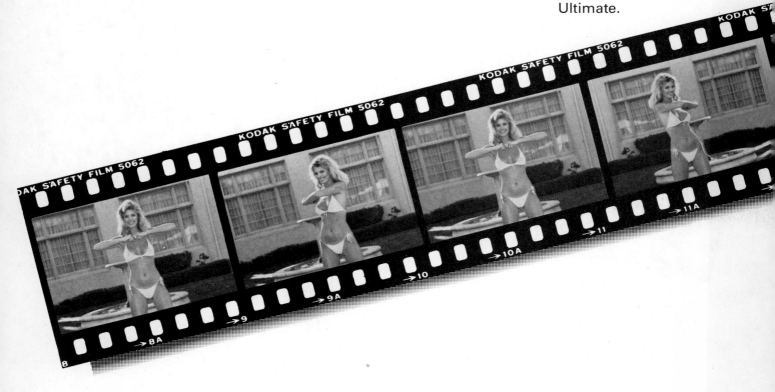

Stretches:

Side and Single Side

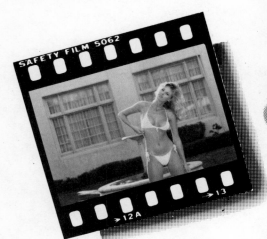

REPS: 20x's each

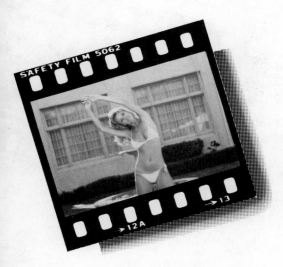

Over Head and Single Over Head

REPS: 20x's each

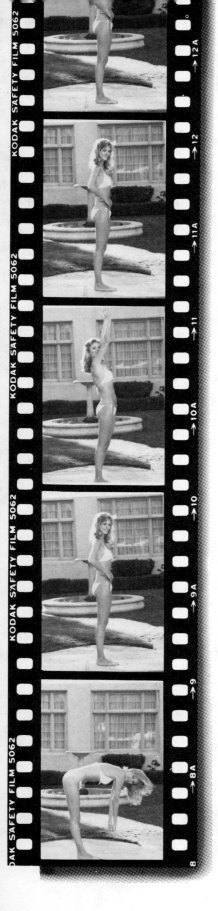

Toe Touches

REPS: 35x's

Hips and up, hips and down, hips and up, hips and down, hip, hip, hooray!

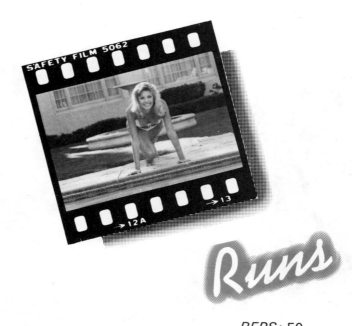

Runs

REPS: 50

Giddy-up!

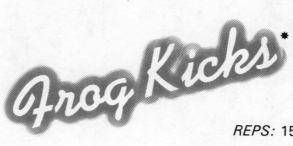

*Frog Kicks**

REPS: 15x's

These are the same Frog Kicks tha
you do when you're swimming b
don't worry if you don't know how
to swim...you're gonna be holdin
on to the edge of the pool.

1. *With your back to the side of th
pool, grasp the edge with both
hands, extend legs straight out.*

2. *With the soles of your feet together, slowly bring knees to
chest.*

3. *Straighten legs from the knees.*

   *Return legs to starting position
   and repeat.*

Do this exercise as fast as you can

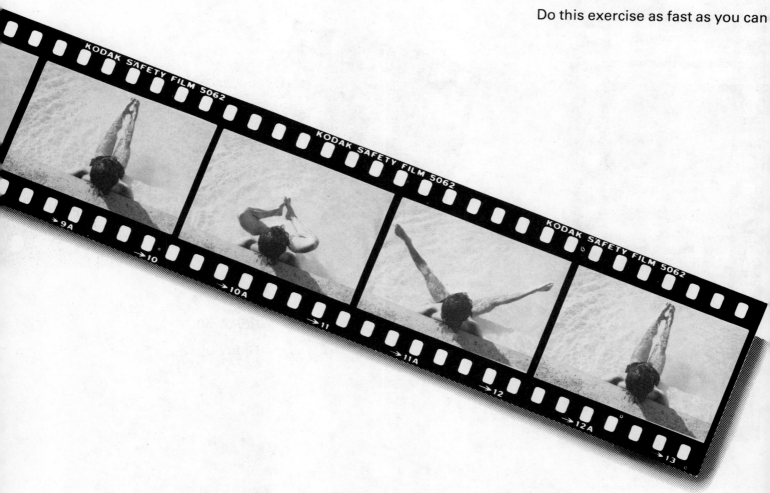

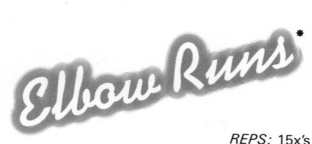

Elbow Runs *

* New exercise.

REPS: 15x's

1. With back against side of pool, elbows resting on pool edge and hands grasping the edge.

2. With legs extended straight out in front gimme Underwater Baby Runs.

Okay, everybody out of the pool! And grab a towel.

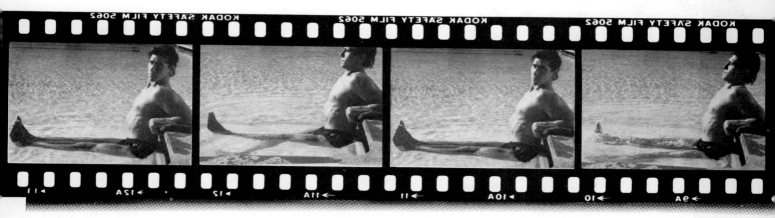

Towel Pulls

*

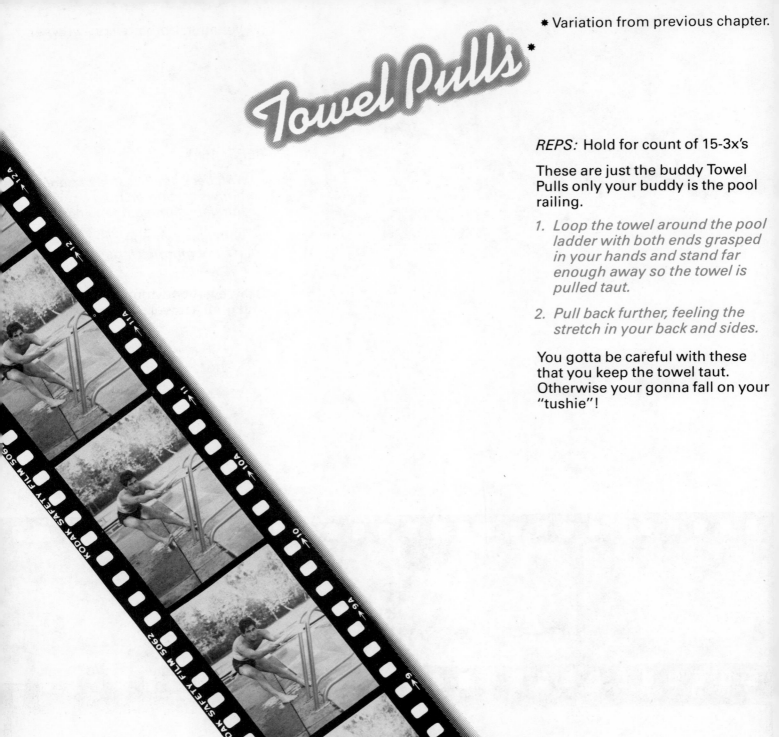

REPS: Hold for count of 15-3x's

These are just the buddy Towel Pulls only your buddy is the pool railing.

1. *Loop the towel around the pool ladder with both ends grasped in your hands and stand far enough away so the towel is pulled taut.*

2. *Pull back further, feeling the stretch in your back and sides.*

You gotta be careful with these that you keep the towel taut. Otherwise your gonna fall on your "tushie"!

Pool Push-Ups

* Variation from previous chapter.

*

REPS: 15x's

You have a choice with these or, if you're truly ambitious, you can do both.

The first kind use the ladder at the pool steps and the second one uses the steps themselves and you stay in the water!

* Variation from previous chapter.

Pool Ladder Push-Ups

REPS: 15x's

1. *Take the Big Boy Push-up position with your toes touching the ground and each hand on one side of the pool step rail.*

2. *Lower to the position shown and then push-up to starting position.*

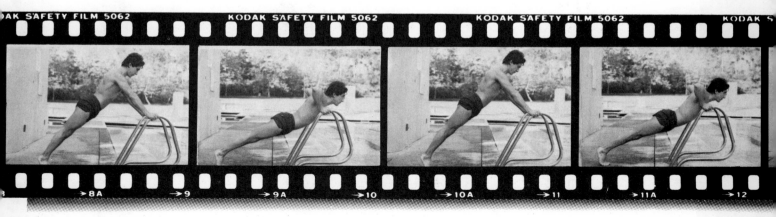

Pool Edge Push-Ups *

FOR: Strengthening upper body
REPS: 15x's

1. While supported by hands in push-up position on pool edge, extend body out in the water.

2. Keeping body held tight, raise and lower yourself on the pool edge.

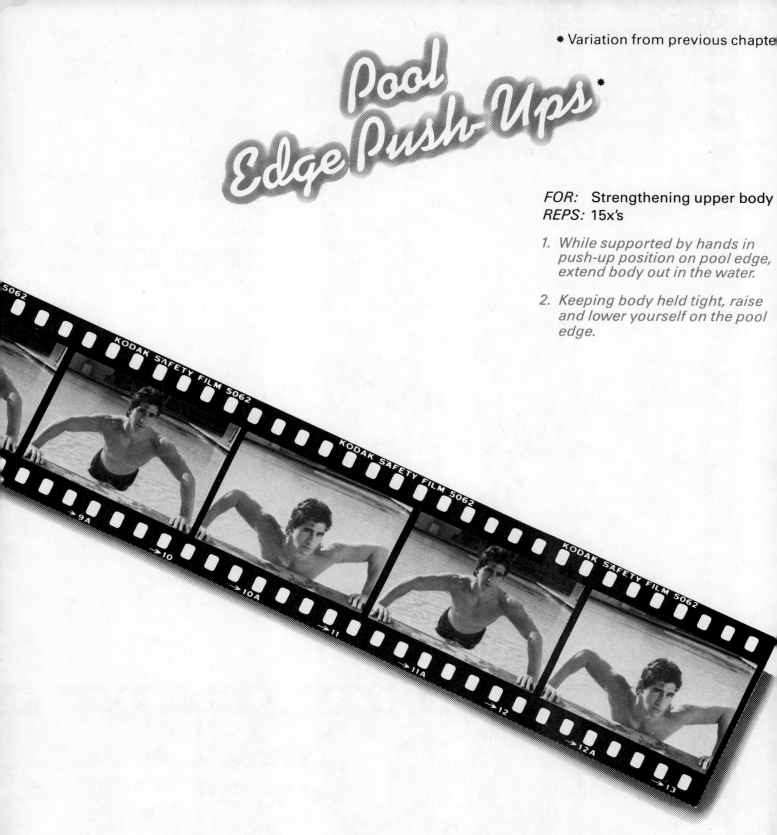

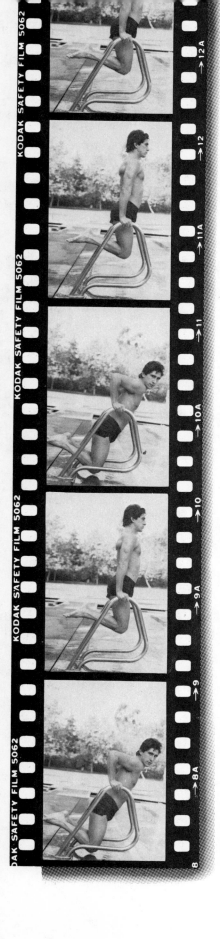

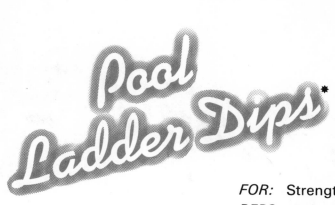

* New exercise.

Pool Ladder Dips*

FOR: Strengthening upper body

REPS: 15x's

1. Support body between pool step rail with straight arms and legs bent at knees.

2. Slowly lower body as far as comfortable without touching the ground while keeping legs bent then return to starting position.

Inverted Curl Pull-Ups

* New exercise.

REPS: 15x's

1. *Come up under the diving board and clasp the side edges with both hands.*

2. *Pull yourself up and return to starting position.*

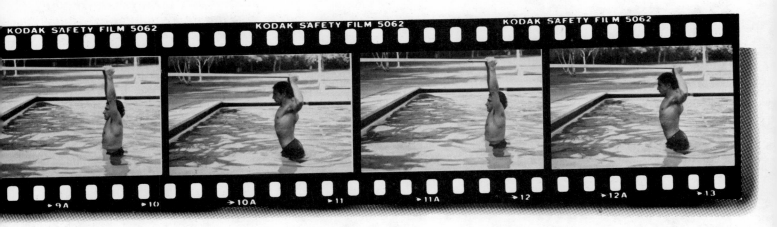

Diving Board Pull-Ups

* New exercise.

REPS: 10x's

These are sort of a reverse Door Knob Curl...sort of but not really.

1. *Come up directly under the front edge of the diving board. Clasp the board with both hands on the front edge.*

2. *Raise and lower yourself keeping your legs extended.*

One more and you can order room service or go lie in the sun.

Treading Water With Arm Swings

REPS: 20x's

Everybody can tread water whether you swim or not! If you don't swim I would suggest that you try this in the shallow end of the pool! But, the water has to be at least shoulder level.

1. With arms extended and hands cupped, move your legs back and forth as in Baby Runs while swinging your arms back and forth with your hands scooping the water for resistance.

That's it! You're a water baby! Now if you decided you didn't want to work out at the hotel pool because you're in Fargo, North Dakota and it's 20 degrees below don't think you're gonna get out of working out! I got a mini-workout guaranteed to get you as wet as if you'd worked out in the pool!

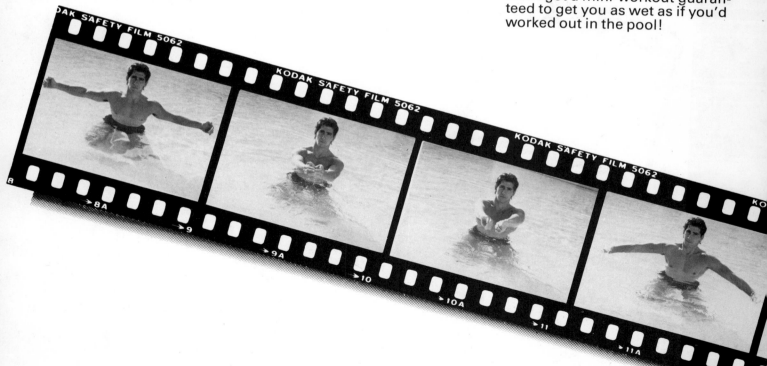

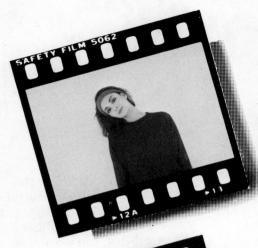

10 *Head Rolls*

REPS: 5x's each direction

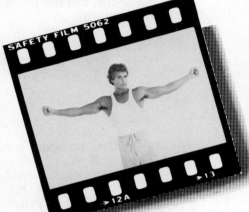

10 *Arm Circles*

REPS: 10x's each direction

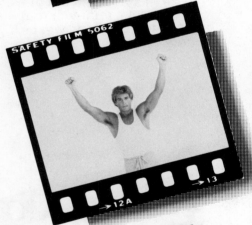

10 *Wheel Rolls*

REPS: 10x's each direction

These are the same as the Wheel
Rolls in Chapter 5 (page 154).
Swing your arms in BIG
circles from the shoulders.

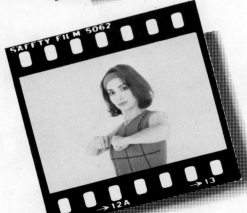

10 *Twisters*

REPS: 1 count 10x's side to side

Stretches:

10 Side

REPS: 10x's each side

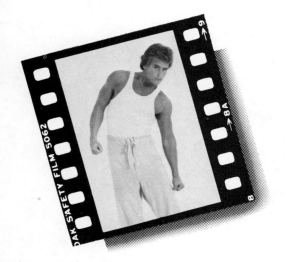

10 Single Side

REPS: 10x's each side

10 Over Head

REPS: 10x's each side

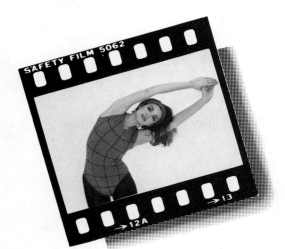

10 Count Single Over Head

REPS: 1 each side held for 10 counts

10 Toe Touches

REPS: 10x's hips and up, hip and down

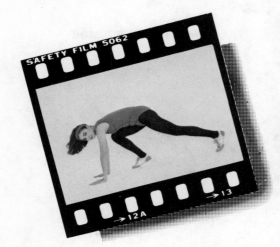

10 Runs

REPS: 10x's

10 Body Burners

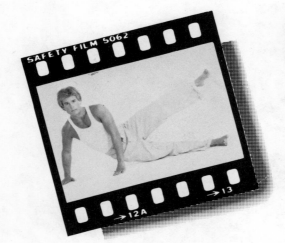

REPS: 10x's

1. *Lie on your side, supporting your weight on hands with straight arms like on page 129.*

2. *Raise and lower upper leg with flexed foot while staying supported by arms.*

   Gimme 25 smokers on each side.

Now stay down there and run!

10 Runs

REPS: 10x's

10 Push-Ups Off Beds

REPS: 10x's

These are a combination of knee Push-ups and two chair Push-ups.

1. Put knees on the edge of bed with hands on floor shoulder width apart.

2. Bending elbows, lower chest and chin to floor.

   Push back up to starting position.

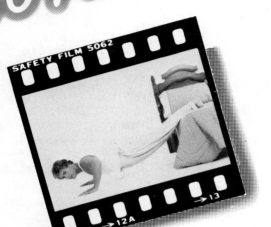

10 Runs

REPS: 10x's

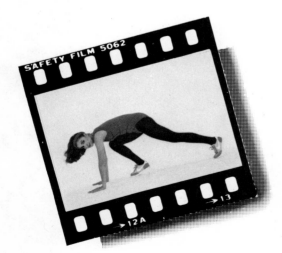

10 Sit Ups / Feet Under Bed

REPS: 10x's

Bet you didn't know all the things a bed could be good for.

1. *Sit on floor with knees bent, feet hooked under bed and arms crossed over chest.*

2. *Lower yourself halfway back and return to starting position.*

   Remember to keep those "Abba- Dabbas" tight!

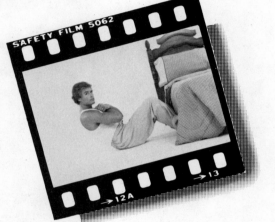

10 Runs

REPS: 10x's

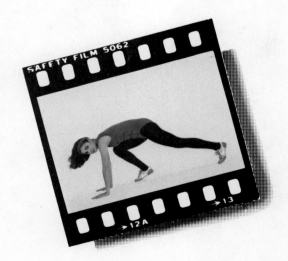

10 Leg Raises

REPS: 10x's each position

Well, you got three different arm positions you have learned with leg raises: hands under "tushies," up on elbows or up on hands. Guess which one I suggest!

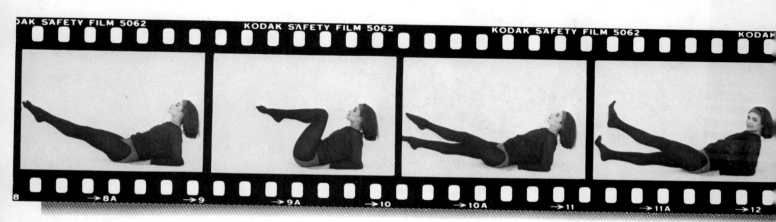

In / Outs

1. Lie on your back propped up on your elbows (aha!) here we go.

2. Bring your knees in to your chest and push them straight out again.

3. Repeat by pulling knees up to chest again and pushing out.

4. Gimme a smokin' 10 and go on to Scissors as shown. Don't let your feet touch the floor during or between the exercises!

Scissors

1. Next 10: legs extended straight out parallel to the floor and held tight.

2. Cross your legs back and forth, for 15 and, GET TOUGH!

Baby Runs

1. Last 20: holding legs straight and TIGHT, flutter stiff legs in tiny runs for 15 counts.

Think this exercise couldn't get any harder?...wait and see!

209

10 Count Wishbone Stretches

REPS: Hold 10 counts left, right, center.

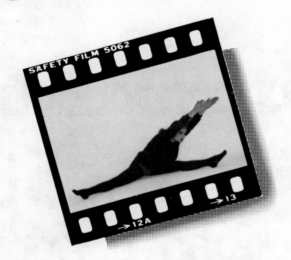

10 Count Hurdles

REPS: Hold for 10 counts each leg.

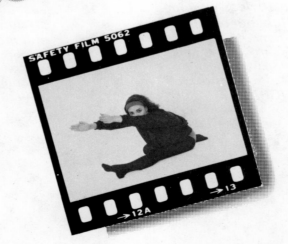

How'd ya do???!!! Did it take ya 10 minutes? It should have. Did you do ten of everything???!!! Did you sweat off ten pounds??? Did the man at the hotel desk call up and tell you to pack your bag and be out in 10 minutes???!!!

Well, sit back and relax. You're in for another smokin,' psyched out, truly hot 10 minutes. Jake "The Snake" Steinfeld wants to "share" something with you and you deserve it since you've come all this way!

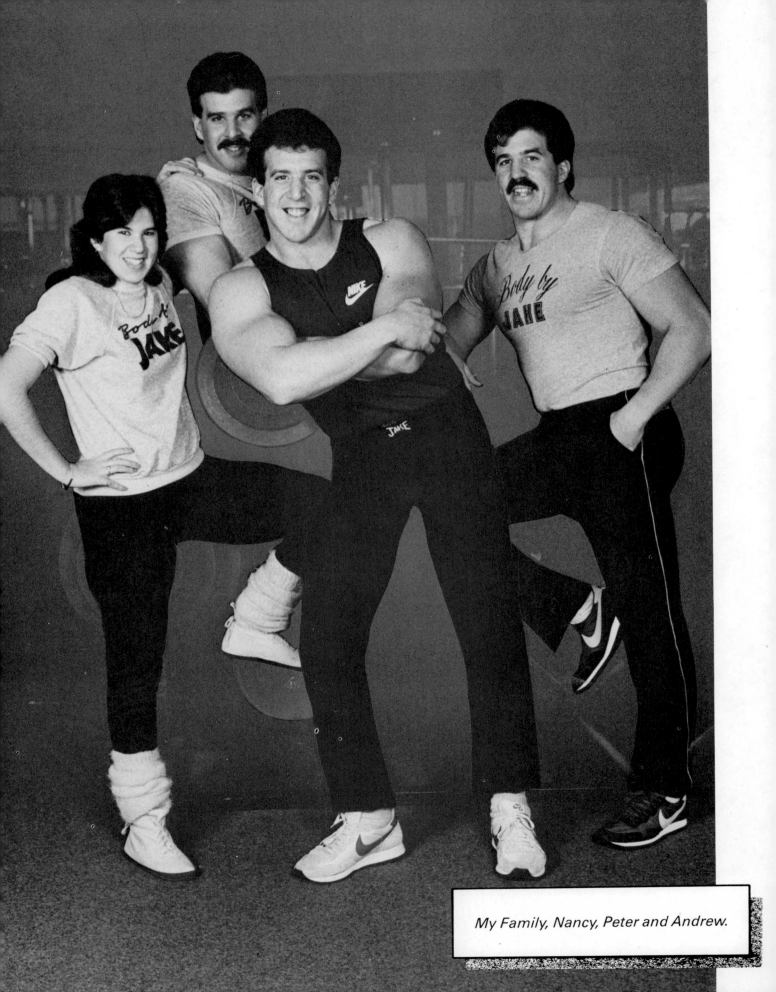

My Family, Nancy, Peter and Andrew.

Chapter Eight

"BODY OF JAKE"

This is it. I gotta talk about it because it's what a lot of you want to know about. It might even be why a lot of you bought the book.

Body of Jake.

I'm real proud of my body and I've been working six days a week for six years to get it like this! No, I didn't always look like this.

I've always wanted to be an entrepreneur. I've always wanted to be cool. (Notice "attitude" and hand in pocket.) There was always something telling me to push on. Then something started telling me that "push" wasn't the right word and maybe it should be "pump."

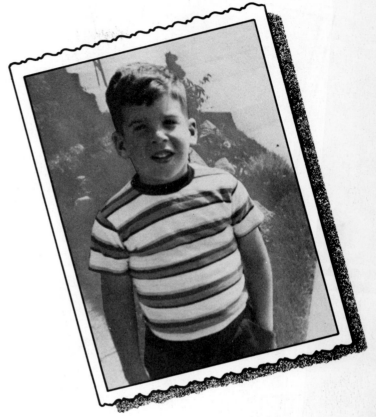

I told my parents about these feelings and they were behind me 100%. My Mom and Dad have always been right there for me. My brothers Andrew and Peter and my sister, Nancy, would have been there for me too but they weren't born yet. Anyway, my folks got me something to pump. Yup, a tricycle. We didn't know there was anything else to "pump" so it was a start.

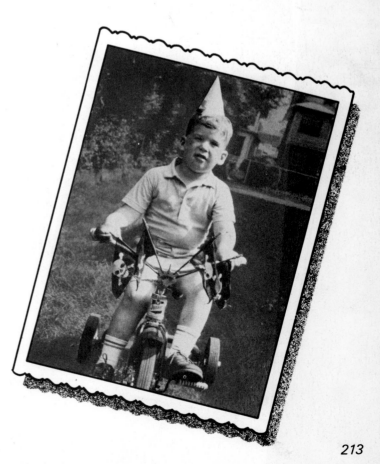

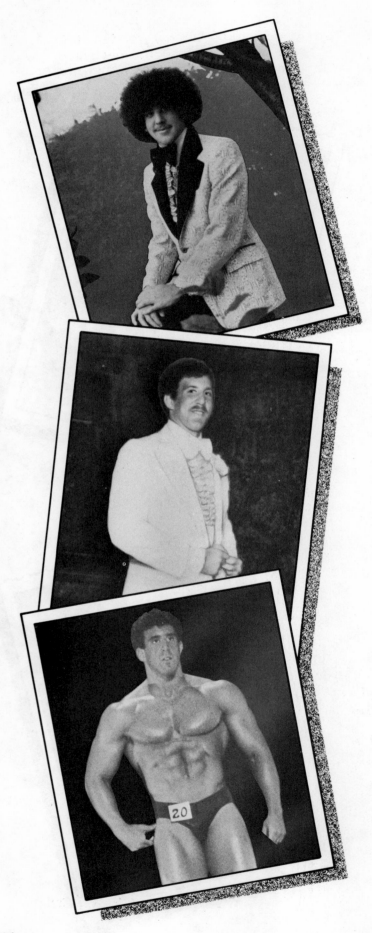

Pumpin' my trike and later my bike kept me happy through my childhood. But, as I grew older I wanted to pump something else. I just wasn't sure what. My folks thought maybe I should get a job in a gas station. I knew that wasn't the answer. So, in the meantime I figured I'd pump whatever was available. Unfortunately it was my hair. Obviously that wasn't the answer either.

In the meantime I got into sports. It distracted me from my preoccupation and it also forced me to deflate my hair!

The next thing I knew I was in college. Anyone who says a college education isn't important is wrong. It was in college that I "found" what to pump! I wanted to pump iron! And, that's where it started. I had found what was for me. Ever since that moment six years ago it's been my life and my work.

Everything I've told you throughout this book is what I truly believe in and live by. I'm not saying that training six days a week at four in the morning is for everyone. But if I'm gonna see my first client at 6 am—I gotta take care of myself first! If I didn't I wouldn't have the strength or the stamina to train 15 clients every day, be in movies, be on TV and radio shows and . . . write a book for you guys.

So now, I'm gonna show you some pieces of my workout. And just remember, you're supposed to be sitting there relaxing. I don't want any of you to EVER, EVER attempt any part of my workout! It's my workout, designed for me and to be done only by me. But, if you decide you want to work with heavy weights, you hire yourself a trainer to come to your house or you go to the gym!

My program is broken down into body parts. Why? Because that's the way I like to work out—that's why! But, no matter what routine I'm doing, every day I warm-up and work my calves and "abs" (you remember those, don't you?).

Here we go!

Mondays and Thursdays
Body parts: Chest and Trimens

I'll first show you something I might start with to work my calves. These are called Donkey Calf Raises.

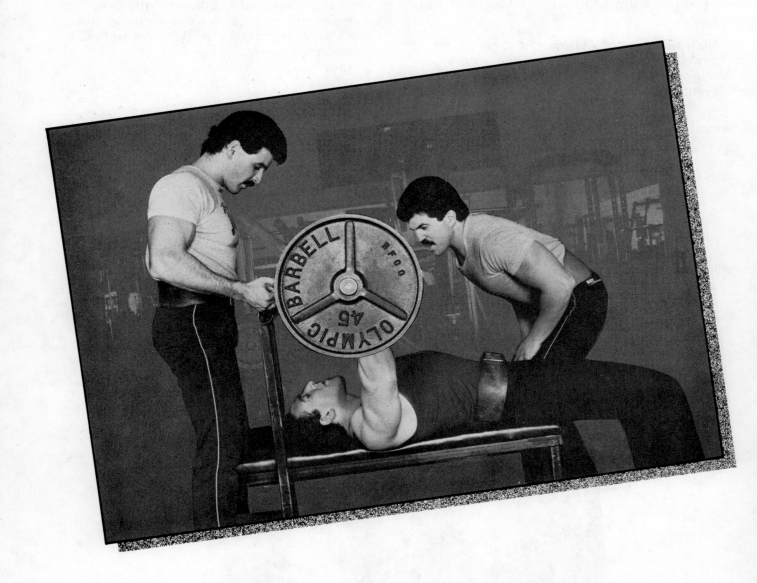

Now I'll show you one of my chest exercises from this program. It's called a Bench Press. You and I *never* did Bench Presses because it requires special equipment *and* a "spotter". These spotters in the picture are special too. They're my brothers Peter and Andrew.

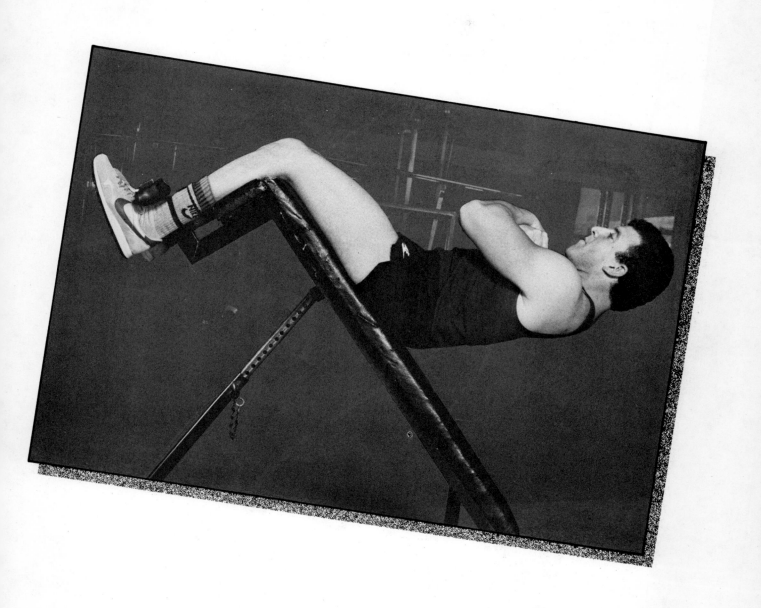

Tuesdays and Fridays
Body parts: Back and Bimens
First let me show you inverted sit ups for my "abs" before the back bimens.

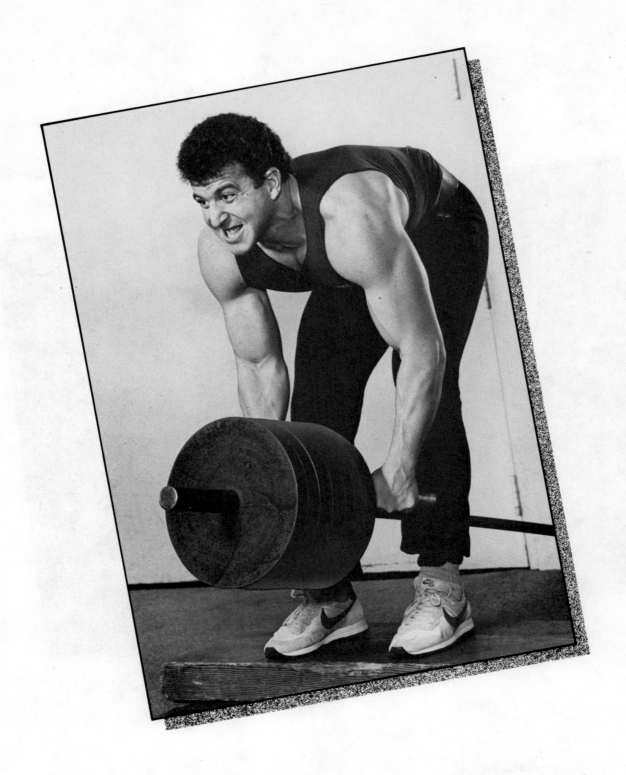

Now, here's one of the exercises I do for my back. I'll show you bimens on Fridays. Anyway, this is called a T-Bar Row and it requires professional equipment and spotters, of course!

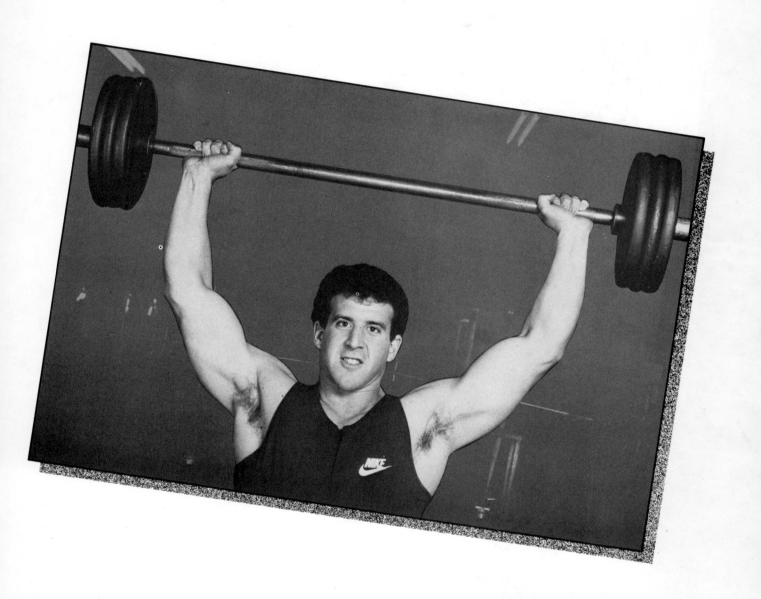

Wednesday—Saturday
Body parts: Shoulders and Legs
Standing dumbbell press.
These are for my shoulders. Don't think these are the same I gave you in an earlier workout.
They aren't!!!!!

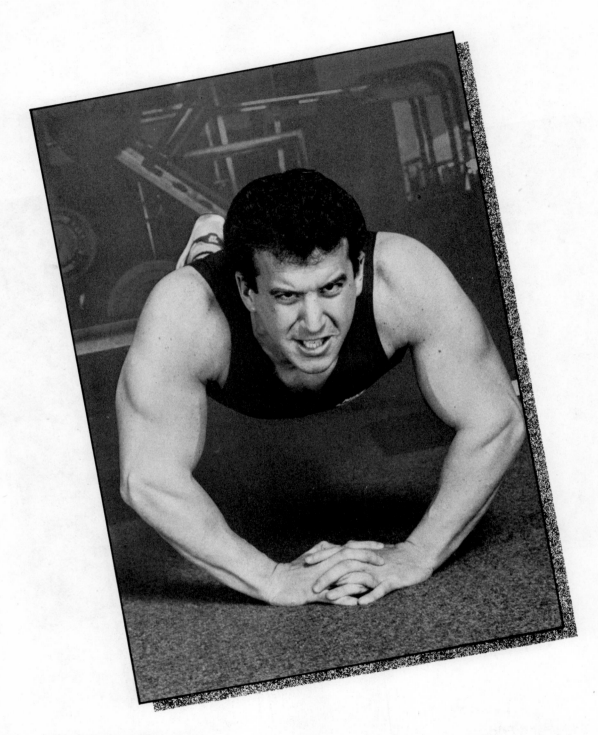

Mondays and Thursdays
Body parts: Chest and Trimens

I already showed you the bench press for the chest so now I'm gonna show you something for my trimens.

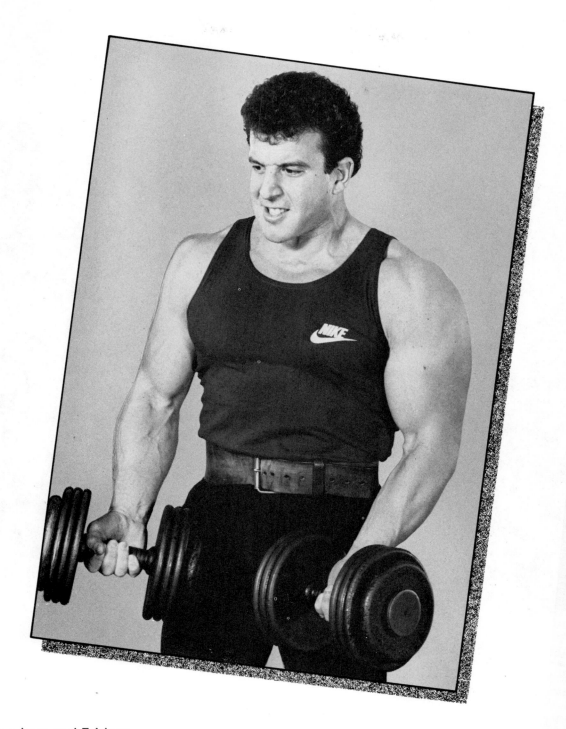

Tuesdays and Fridays
Body parts: Back and Bimens

You saw the T-Bar Row for my back and everyday I do those T-Bar Rows I also do standing dumbbell curls for ... guess!

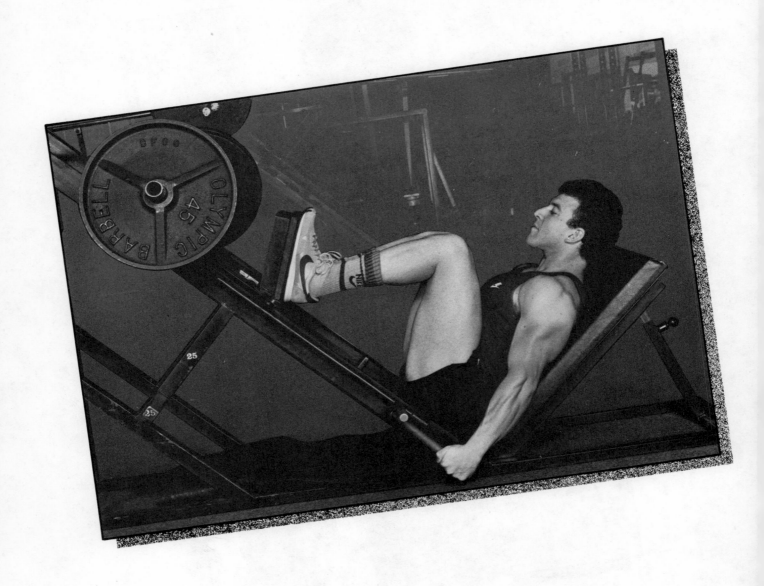

Wednesday—Saturday
Body parts: Shoulders and Legs

I don't know about you but I can't wait for Sunday! I showed you shoulders and now you get legs! This is called a Leg Press.

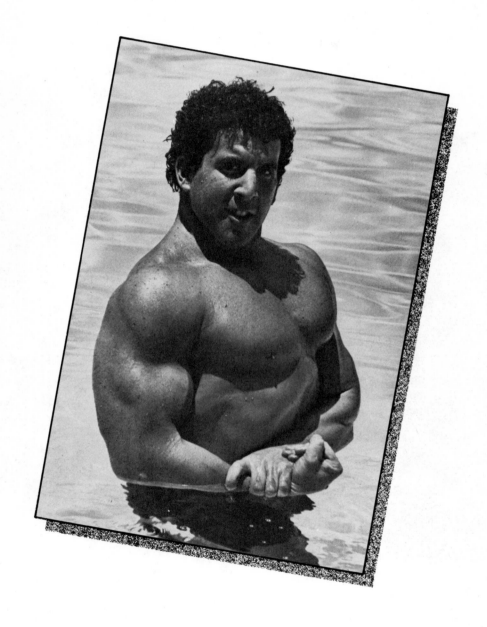

Sunday!!
Body parts: everything!!

"DON'T QUIT"

When things go wrong as they sometimes will,
When the road you're trudging seems all uphill,
When the funds are low and the debts are high
And you want to smile, but you have to sigh,
When care is pressing you down a bit
Rest, if you must, but don't you quit.
Life is queer with its twists and turns
As every one of us sometimes learns
And many a failure turns about
When he might have won had he stuck it out;
Don't give up though the pace seems slow—
You may succeed with another blow,
Success is failure turned inside out—
The silver tint of the clouds of doubt,
And you never can tell how close you are,
It may be near when it seems so far;
So stick to the fight when you're hardest hit—
It's when things seem worst that you must not quit

Anonymous—

Remember: You can't quit if you don't begin!

LET'S KEEP HUSTLING!!!!!!